PNEUMONIA AND ASTHMA
Natural Home Remedies

Dr. Harry Rusden

Copyright © 2024 Dr. Harry Rusden
Alright reserved

Table of Contents

I. **Introduction to Pneumonia and Asthma**
   A. Understanding Pneumonia
   B. Understanding Asthma
   C. Differentiating Between Pneumonia and Asthma
   D. Importance of Natural Remedies

II. **Lifestyle Changes for Managing Pneumonia and Asthma**
   A. Diet Modifications
   B. Exercise and Physical Activity Recommendations
   C. Environmental Adjustments
   D. Stress Management Techniques

III. **Herbal Remedies for Pneumonia and Asthma**
   A. Eucalyptus
   B. Ginger
   C. Turmeric
   D. Licorice Root
   E. Ginseng

IV. **Essential Oils for Respiratory Health**
   A. Peppermint Oil
   B. Tea Tree Oil

   C. Lavender Oil
   D. Eucalyptus Oil
   E. Oregano Oil

V. **Homeopathic Remedies for Pneumonia and Asthma**
   A. Antimonium Tartaricum
   B. Arsenicum Album
   C. Bryonia
   D. Ipecacuanha
   E. Spongia Tosta

VI. **Dietary Supplements for Respiratory Support**
   A. Vitamin C
   B. Vitamin D
   C. Magnesium
   D. Omega-3 Fatty Acids
   E. Quercetin

VII. **Breathing Exercises and Techniques**
   A. Diaphragmatic Breathing
   B. Pursed Lip Breathing
   C. Buteyko Breathing Technique
   D. Yoga and Pranayama

VIII. **Steam Therapy and Humidification**
   A. Steam Inhalation

   B. Humidifiers and Vaporizers
   C. Herbal Steam Blends

IX. **Acupuncture and Acupressure Points for Respiratory Health**
   A. Lung Meridian Points
   B. Conception Vessel Meridian Points
   C. Governing Vessel Meridian Points

X. **Precautions and Considerations**
   A. Consultation with Healthcare Provider
   B. Allergic Reactions and Sensitivities
   C. Monitoring Symptoms
   D. Integration with Conventional Treatment

XI. **Conclusion**
   A. Recap of Natural Remedies for Pneumonia and Asthma
   B. Importance of Personalized Approach
   C. Long-Term Management Strategies

Chapter 1

Introduction to Pneumonia and Asthma

Pneumonia and asthma are both respiratory conditions that can significantly impact an individual's quality of life. Understanding these conditions is crucial for effective management and treatment.

Pneumonia is an infection that inflames the air sacs in one or both lungs, filling them with fluid or pus, leading to symptoms such as cough, fever, difficulty breathing, and chest pain. It can range from mild to severe and can be caused by bacteria, viruses, or fungi. Pneumonia can be particularly dangerous for young children, the elderly, and individuals with weakened immune systems.

Asthma, on the other hand, is a chronic inflammatory condition of the airways characterized by episodes of wheezing, breathlessness, chest tightness, and coughing, especially at night or early in the morning. Asthma attacks can be triggered by various factors, including allergens, irritants, respiratory infections, exercise, and stress. While asthma cannot be cured, it can be effectively managed with proper treatment and lifestyle modifications.

Both pneumonia and asthma require careful management to prevent complications and improve respiratory function. In this guide, we will explore natural remedies and lifestyle changes that can help alleviate symptoms and support overall respiratory health for individuals dealing with these conditions.

Understanding Pneumonia

Pneumonia is a common respiratory infection characterized by inflammation of the air sacs in the lungs. This inflammation can be caused by various infectious agents, including bacteria, viruses, and fungi. Understanding the key aspects of pneumonia is essential for recognizing its symptoms, diagnosing the condition, and initiating appropriate treatment.

1. **Causes**: Pneumonia can be caused by different pathogens, with the most common being bacteria and viruses. Bacterial pneumonia is often associated with Streptococcus pneumoniae, while viral pneumonia can be caused by influenza viruses, respiratory syncytial virus (RSV), and others.

Fungal pneumonia is less common and typically affects individuals with weakened immune systems.

2. **Transmission**: Pneumonia-causing pathogens can be transmitted through respiratory droplets from coughing, sneezing, or close contact with an infected person. Certain risk factors, such as advanced age, weakened immune system, chronic lung diseases, and smoking, can increase susceptibility to pneumonia.

3. **Symptoms**: Common symptoms of pneumonia include cough (with or without sputum production), fever, chills, difficulty breathing, chest pain, fatigue, and confusion, especially in older adults. Symptoms may vary depending on the severity of the infection and the underlying cause.

4. **Diagnosis**: Diagnosis of pneumonia typically involves a combination of clinical evaluation, physical examination, and diagnostic tests. These may include chest X-rays, blood tests (such as complete blood count and blood cultures), sputum analysis, and sometimes more advanced imaging studies or respiratory tests.

5. **Treatment**: Treatment for pneumonia depends on the cause and severity of the infection. Bacterial

pneumonia is often treated with antibiotics, while antiviral medications may be used for viral pneumonia. Supportive care measures, such as rest, adequate hydration, and fever management, are also important. In severe cases, hospitalization and intravenous antibiotics may be necessary.

6. **Prevention**: Preventive measures for pneumonia include vaccination against common pathogens, such as the pneumococcal vaccine and the influenza vaccine. Good hygiene practices, such as regular handwashing, covering coughs and sneezes, and avoiding close contact with sick individuals, can also help reduce the risk of infection.

Understanding pneumonia and its various aspects is crucial for early recognition, prompt treatment, and prevention of complications. Individuals with symptoms suggestive of pneumonia should seek medical attention for proper evaluation and management.

Understanding Asthma

Asthma is a chronic inflammatory respiratory condition characterized by reversible airway obstruction, bronchial hyperresponsiveness, and recurrent episodes of wheezing, breathlessness, chest tightness, and coughing. Understanding the key aspects of asthma is crucial for effective management and improving quality of life for individuals living with this condition.

1. **Pathophysiology**:
   - Asthma involves inflammation of the airways, leading to swelling and narrowing of the bronchial tubes. This inflammation is triggered by various stimuli, including allergens, irritants, respiratory infections, exercise, and stress. In response to these triggers, the airways become hyperreactive, leading to bronchoconstriction and symptoms of asthma.

2. **Symptoms**:
   - Common symptoms of asthma include wheezing (a whistling or squeaky sound when breathing), breathlessness, chest tightness, and coughing, especially at night or early in the morning. Symptoms may vary in severity and frequency from person to person and can range from mild to severe, potentially leading to asthma attacks or exacerbations.

3. **Triggers**:
   - Asthma symptoms can be triggered by a wide range of factors, including:
     - Allergens (such as pollen, dust mites, pet dander)
     - Irritants (such as smoke, pollution, strong odors)
     - Respiratory infections (such as colds, flu)
     - Exercise or physical activity
     - Changes in weather or temperature
     - Emotional stress or anxiety

4. **Diagnosis**:
   - Diagnosis of asthma involves a comprehensive evaluation of symptoms, medical history, physical examination, and pulmonary function tests. Lung function tests, such as spirometry and peak flow measurements, help assess airflow obstruction and bronchial responsiveness. Allergy testing and imaging studies may be performed to rule out other conditions or identify specific triggers.

5. **Treatment**:
   - Treatment for asthma aims to control symptoms, prevent exacerbations, and improve lung function. This typically involves a combination of medication and lifestyle modifications, including:

- **Controller Medications**: Inhaled corticosteroids, long-acting beta-agonists, leukotriene modifiers, and biologic therapies help reduce inflammation and prevent asthma symptoms.
- **Rescue Medications**: Short-acting beta-agonists (such as albuterol) provide quick relief of asthma symptoms during flare-ups or asthma attacks.
- **Allergy Management**: Identifying and avoiding allergens that trigger asthma symptoms can help reduce the frequency and severity of asthma exacerbations.
- **Asthma Action Plan**: Developing a personalized asthma action plan in collaboration with a healthcare provider helps patients recognize and manage asthma symptoms effectively, including when to adjust medication doses or seek medical attention.

6. **Lifestyle Management**:
   - Lifestyle modifications, such as maintaining a healthy weight, staying physically active, avoiding tobacco smoke, managing stress, and improving indoor air quality, can help support overall asthma management and reduce the risk of exacerbations.

7. **Monitoring and Follow-Up**:
   - Regular monitoring of asthma symptoms, lung function, and medication adherence is essential for adjusting treatment as needed and preventing asthma exacerbations. Healthcare providers may recommend periodic follow-up visits to assess asthma control, review treatment goals, and update the asthma action plan.

By understanding the underlying mechanisms, triggers, diagnosis, and management strategies for asthma, individuals with this condition can better control their symptoms and lead active, healthy lives with proper medical guidance and support.

Differentiating Between Pneumonia and Asthma

Pneumonia and asthma are two distinct respiratory conditions with different underlying causes, symptoms, and management approaches. Understanding the key differences between them is essential for accurate diagnosis and appropriate treatment.

1. **Underlying Cause**:
   - Pneumonia: Pneumonia is primarily caused by infection with bacteria, viruses, or fungi that lead to inflammation and fluid buildup in the air sacs of the lungs.
   - Asthma: Asthma is a chronic inflammatory condition of the airways, often triggered by allergens, irritants, respiratory infections, exercise, or stress. It is not primarily infectious like pneumonia.

2. **Symptoms**:
   - Pneumonia: Common symptoms of pneumonia include cough (with or without sputum production), fever, chills, difficulty breathing, chest pain, fatigue, and confusion. Symptoms may develop suddenly and are typically more severe than those of asthma.
   - Asthma: Symptoms of asthma include wheezing, breathlessness, chest tightness, and coughing, particularly at night or early in the morning. Asthma symptoms may vary in intensity and frequency and can be triggered by specific environmental factors.

3. **Onset and Duration**:
   - Pneumonia: Pneumonia often presents with acute onset of symptoms, progressing rapidly over a

few days. Without prompt treatment, pneumonia symptoms can worsen quickly and may require hospitalization.

- Asthma: Asthma symptoms can develop gradually or suddenly (asthma attack) and may persist over a longer period. Asthma is a chronic condition that requires ongoing management to prevent exacerbations and maintain respiratory function.

4. **Diagnostic Tests**:
   - Pneumonia: Diagnosis of pneumonia typically involves a combination of clinical evaluation, physical examination, and diagnostic tests, including chest X-rays, blood tests, and sputum analysis.
   - Asthma: Diagnosis of asthma involves assessing symptoms, lung function tests (such as spirometry), and sometimes allergy testing or imaging studies to rule out other conditions.

5. **Treatment Approach**:
   - Pneumonia: Treatment for pneumonia often includes antibiotics for bacterial infections, antiviral medications for viral infections, and supportive care measures such as rest, hydration, and fever management.

- Asthma: Treatment for asthma focuses on controlling inflammation and bronchoconstriction with medications such as inhaled corticosteroids, bronchodilators, and oral medications. Asthma management also involves identifying and avoiding triggers and maintaining a personalized asthma action plan.

By understanding the differences between pneumonia and asthma in terms of their causes, symptoms, and management, healthcare providers can accurately diagnose and treat these respiratory conditions, improving patient outcomes and quality of life.

Importance of Natural Remedies

Natural remedies play a significant role in managing various health conditions, including respiratory ailments like asthma and pneumonia. Understanding the importance of natural remedies can help individuals make informed choices about their healthcare and complement conventional treatments effectively. Here are several reasons why natural remedies are valuable:

1. **Reduced Side Effects**: Many natural remedies, such as herbal supplements, essential oils, and dietary changes, have fewer side effects compared to pharmaceutical medications. This can be particularly beneficial for individuals who are sensitive to or experience adverse reactions from conventional treatments.

2. **Holistic Approach**: Natural remedies often address the underlying factors contributing to health conditions rather than just alleviating symptoms. They promote a holistic approach to wellness by supporting the body's natural healing processes and overall health.

3. **Supportive Care**: Natural remedies can serve as supportive care measures to enhance the effectiveness of conventional treatments. For respiratory conditions like asthma and pneumonia, natural remedies can help alleviate symptoms, reduce inflammation, and support respiratory function alongside prescribed medications.

4. **Accessibility and Affordability**: Many natural remedies are readily available and accessible, often at a lower cost than prescription medications. This accessibility makes natural remedies an attractive option for individuals

seeking alternative or complementary treatments, especially in regions with limited access to healthcare resources.

5. **Personalized Treatment Options**: Natural remedies offer a wide range of treatment options that can be tailored to individual preferences and needs. From dietary modifications to herbal supplements to breathing exercises, individuals can choose natural remedies that align with their lifestyle, beliefs, and health goals.

6. **Empowerment and Self-Care**: Incorporating natural remedies into a healthcare routine empowers individuals to take an active role in their health and well-being. Learning about natural remedies and self-care practices fosters a sense of empowerment and self-efficacy in managing health conditions.

7. **Preventive Health Benefits**: Many natural remedies not only help alleviate symptoms but also promote overall health and prevent future health issues. For example, dietary changes that focus on anti-inflammatory foods can support respiratory health and reduce the risk of exacerbations for individuals with asthma or pneumonia.

8. **Cultural and Traditional Wisdom**: Natural remedies often draw from cultural and traditional healing practices that have been passed down through generations. These remedies reflect a wealth of knowledge and wisdom about the natural world and its potential to promote health and well-being.

In summary, natural remedies offer valuable benefits for individuals seeking alternative or complementary approaches to managing respiratory conditions like asthma and pneumonia. By integrating natural remedies alongside conventional treatments, individuals can optimize their health outcomes and improve their overall quality of life. However, it's essential to consult with healthcare providers before starting any new treatment regimen, especially if you have existing health conditions or are taking medications.

Chapter 2

Lifestyle Changes for Managing Pneumonia and Asthma

Implementing lifestyle changes is an integral part of managing pneumonia and asthma effectively. These changes can help reduce the frequency and severity of symptoms, improve overall respiratory health, and enhance the effectiveness of medical treatments. Here are key lifestyle modifications for managing pneumonia and asthma:

1. **Quit Smoking**: Smoking worsens respiratory conditions and increases the risk of complications. Quitting smoking is crucial for improving lung function, reducing inflammation, and lowering the risk of pneumonia and asthma exacerbations.

2. **Avoid Secondhand Smoke**: Exposure to secondhand smoke can trigger asthma symptoms and increase the risk of respiratory infections. Minimize exposure to smoke from cigarettes, cigars, or other tobacco products, especially in indoor environments.

3. **Maintain a Healthy Weight**: Obesity and excess weight can worsen asthma symptoms and

increase the risk of complications from pneumonia. Adopting a balanced diet and regular exercise routine can help achieve and maintain a healthy weight, improve lung function, and enhance overall health.

4. **Follow a Balanced Diet**: A nutritious diet rich in fruits, vegetables, whole grains, and lean proteins provides essential nutrients and antioxidants that support respiratory health and immune function. Avoiding processed foods, excessive sugar, and unhealthy fats can help reduce inflammation and strengthen the body's defenses against respiratory infections.

5. **Stay Hydrated**: Adequate hydration is essential for maintaining healthy mucus membranes and facilitating mucus clearance from the airways. Drink plenty of water throughout the day to stay hydrated and promote respiratory health.

6. **Manage Stress**: Stress can exacerbate asthma symptoms and weaken the immune system, increasing susceptibility to respiratory infections like pneumonia. Practice stress-reduction techniques such as deep breathing exercises, meditation, yoga, or mindfulness to manage stress effectively and promote relaxation.

7. **Get Regular Exercise**: Regular physical activity strengthens the respiratory muscles, improves lung function, and enhances overall cardiovascular health. Engage in aerobic exercises such as walking, swimming, cycling, or jogging to promote respiratory fitness and reduce the risk of asthma exacerbations.

8. **Practice Good Hygiene**: Practicing good hygiene habits, such as regular handwashing with soap and water, helps prevent the spread of respiratory infections like pneumonia. Avoid close contact with individuals who have respiratory symptoms, and cover your mouth and nose when coughing or sneezing to reduce the transmission of infectious droplets.

9. **Maintain Indoor Air Quality**: Indoor air pollutants such as dust, pet dander, mold, and volatile organic compounds (VOCs) can trigger asthma symptoms and worsen respiratory health. Use air purifiers, maintain a clean living environment, and minimize exposure to indoor allergens to improve indoor air quality.

10. **Follow Medical Recommendations**: Adhere to prescribed medications, treatment plans, and follow-up appointments recommended by

healthcare providers for managing pneumonia and asthma. Communicate any concerns or changes in symptoms promptly to ensure timely intervention and appropriate management.

By incorporating these lifestyle changes into daily routines, individuals can effectively manage pneumonia and asthma, reduce symptom severity, and improve overall respiratory health and quality of life. It's essential to work closely with healthcare providers to develop personalized management plans that address individual needs and preferences.

Diet Modifications for Managing Pneumonia and Asthma

Making dietary modifications can play a significant role in managing pneumonia and asthma by supporting immune function, reducing inflammation, and promoting overall respiratory health. Here are dietary recommendations tailored to managing these respiratory conditions:

1. **Anti-Inflammatory Foods**: Incorporate foods rich in antioxidants and anti-inflammatory nutrients to help reduce inflammation in the

airways and support respiratory health. Examples include:
  - Fruits: Berries (blueberries, strawberries, raspberries), citrus fruits (oranges, lemons, grapefruits), apples, and cherries.
  - Vegetables: Leafy greens (spinach, kale, Swiss chard), cruciferous vegetables (broccoli, Brussels sprouts, cauliflower), bell peppers, and tomatoes.
  - Nuts and Seeds: Almonds, walnuts, flaxseeds, and chia seeds.
  - Fatty Fish: Salmon, mackerel, trout, and sardines, rich in omega-3 fatty acids.

2. **Omega-3 Fatty Acids**: Include sources of omega-3 fatty acids in your diet to help reduce inflammation and support respiratory function. These include fatty fish, flaxseeds, chia seeds, walnuts, and algae-based supplements.

3. **Vitamin D-Rich Foods**: Vitamin D plays a role in immune function and respiratory health. Include foods high in vitamin D, such as fatty fish (salmon, tuna), fortified dairy products, egg yolks, and mushrooms.

4. **Probiotic-Rich Foods**: Probiotics promote gut health and may help modulate the immune system.

Include probiotic-rich foods in your diet, such as yogurt, kefir, sauerkraut, kimchi, and kombucha.

5. **Avoid Food Triggers**: Identify and avoid foods that may trigger asthma symptoms or allergic reactions. Common food triggers include dairy products, gluten, soy, shellfish, and certain food additives or preservatives.

6. **Hydration**: Stay well-hydrated by drinking plenty of water throughout the day. Proper hydration helps maintain optimal mucus production and clearance in the airways, supporting respiratory health.

7. **Limit Processed Foods and Sugary Beverages**: Processed foods and sugary beverages can contribute to inflammation and may exacerbate respiratory symptoms. Minimize intake of processed snacks, sugary drinks, refined grains, and desserts.

8. **Herbal Teas**: Certain herbal teas may have soothing effects on the respiratory system and help alleviate symptoms. Consider drinking herbal teas such as chamomile, ginger, peppermint, and licorice root tea.

9. **Moderate Alcohol Consumption**: Limit alcohol consumption, as excessive alcohol intake can weaken the immune system and exacerbate respiratory conditions. If you choose to drink alcohol, do so in moderation and avoid excessive consumption.

10. **Balanced Meals**: Aim for balanced meals that include a combination of lean proteins, healthy fats, complex carbohydrates, and a variety of fruits and vegetables to ensure adequate nutrient intake and support overall health.

By incorporating these dietary modifications into your lifestyle, you can help manage pneumonia and asthma symptoms, support respiratory health, and enhance overall well-being. It's essential to consult with a healthcare provider or a registered dietitian to develop a personalized dietary plan that meets your specific nutritional needs and addresses any underlying health conditions.

Exercise and Physical Activity for Managing Pneumonia and Asthma

Regular exercise and physical activity play a crucial role in managing pneumonia and asthma by improving respiratory function, strengthening the immune system, and promoting overall health and well-being. However, it's essential to approach exercise cautiously and tailor activities to individual needs and limitations. Here are some guidelines for incorporating exercise and physical activity into a management plan for pneumonia and asthma:

1. **Consult with Healthcare Provider**: Before starting any exercise program, especially for individuals with pneumonia or poorly controlled asthma, it's essential to consult with a healthcare provider. They can provide personalized recommendations based on your current health status, medical history, and fitness level.

2. **Choose Suitable Activities**: Opt for low-impact, moderate-intensity activities that are less likely to trigger asthma symptoms or exacerbate respiratory issues. Examples include walking, swimming, cycling, yoga, tai chi, and gentle stretching exercises.

3. **Warm-Up and Cool Down**: Prior to exercising, perform a thorough warm-up to prepare the body for physical activity and reduce the risk of injury. Similarly, include a cooldown period after

exercising to gradually lower heart rate and prevent post-exercise symptoms.

4. **Monitor Symptoms**: Pay attention to how your body responds to exercise and monitor for any signs of respiratory distress or asthma symptoms. If you experience chest tightness, wheezing, coughing, or shortness of breath during exercise, stop activity immediately and rest.

5. **Use Asthma Medication as Prescribed**: Take prescribed asthma medications, such as bronchodilators or controller medications, as recommended by your healthcare provider before engaging in physical activity. Proper medication management can help prevent exercise-induced asthma symptoms and improve exercise tolerance.

6. **Stay Hydrated**: Drink plenty of water before, during, and after exercise to stay hydrated and maintain optimal respiratory function. Dehydration can exacerbate asthma symptoms and reduce exercise performance.

7. **Avoid Outdoor Allergens**: If outdoor allergens trigger asthma symptoms, such as pollen or air pollution, consider exercising indoors or during times when allergen levels are lower. Use air

purifiers and keep windows closed during high pollen seasons.

8. **Modify Exercise Intensity**: Adjust the intensity and duration of exercise based on individual fitness levels, asthma control, and respiratory health. Start with shorter sessions of low-impact activities and gradually increase intensity and duration as tolerated.

9. **Breathe Through the Nose**: Encourage nasal breathing during exercise, as it helps filter, humidify, and warm incoming air, reducing the likelihood of asthma symptoms triggered by cold or dry air.

10. **Listen to Your Body**: Pay attention to your body's signals and respect its limits. If you experience persistent symptoms or difficulty breathing during exercise, seek medical attention and modify your exercise routine as needed.

By incorporating exercise and physical activity into a comprehensive management plan for pneumonia and asthma, individuals can improve respiratory function, enhance overall fitness, and enjoy a better quality of life. It's essential to work closely with healthcare providers and exercise professionals to develop a safe and effective exercise program tailored to individual needs and goals.

Environmental Adjustments for Managing Pneumonia and Asthma

Making adjustments to the environment can help individuals with pneumonia and asthma reduce exposure to triggers and irritants that worsen symptoms or exacerbate respiratory conditions. By creating a clean and allergen-free environment, individuals can improve respiratory health and minimize the risk of complications. Here are some environmental adjustments to consider:

1. **Allergen Control**:
   - Dust Mites: Use dust-proof covers on pillows and mattresses, wash bedding in hot water weekly, and vacuum carpets and upholstered furniture regularly.
   - Pet Dander: Keep pets out of bedrooms and off furniture, bathe pets regularly, and use air purifiers with HEPA filters to remove pet dander from the air.
   - Mold: Keep humidity levels in the home below 50% to prevent mold growth, fix leaks and water

damage promptly, and use exhaust fans in bathrooms and kitchens.

2. **Indoor Air Quality**:
   - Ventilation: Ensure adequate ventilation in the home by opening windows and using exhaust fans in bathrooms and kitchens to remove indoor pollutants and moisture.
   - Air Purification: Use air purifiers with HEPA filters to remove airborne allergens, pollutants, and irritants from indoor air, especially in bedrooms and living areas.
   - Smoking: Establish a smoke-free environment by prohibiting smoking indoors and encouraging smokers to quit or smoke outside away from windows and doors.

3. **Avoidance of Irritants**:
   - Environmental Tobacco Smoke: Minimize exposure to secondhand smoke by avoiding areas where smoking is allowed and asking family members or visitors to smoke outside.
   - Strong Odors and Chemicals: Use unscented or hypoallergenic cleaning products, avoid strong perfumes or air fresheners, and ventilate areas when painting or using chemicals.

4. **Pollen and Outdoor Allergens**:
   - Pollen: Keep windows and doors closed during high pollen seasons, use air conditioning with pollen filters, and shower and change clothes after spending time outdoors.
   - Air Quality Alerts: Monitor local air quality forecasts and avoid outdoor activities on days when air pollution levels are high, especially during ozone or smog alerts.

5. **Humidity Control**:
   - Humidifiers: Use humidifiers to add moisture to dry indoor air during winter months, but clean and maintain them regularly to prevent mold and bacterial growth.
   - Dehumidifiers: Use dehumidifiers in damp areas such as basements or bathrooms to reduce humidity levels and prevent mold growth.

6. **Bedroom Environment**:
   - Bedding: Use hypoallergenic pillows and bedding materials, wash bedding in hot water weekly, and avoid using down-filled or feather pillows.
   - Flooring: Consider replacing carpeting with hardwood or tile flooring, which is easier to clean and less likely to harbor allergens.

7. **Regular Cleaning and Maintenance**:
   - Vacuuming: Vacuum carpets, rugs, and upholstered furniture regularly using a vacuum cleaner with a HEPA filter to trap dust and allergens.
   - Mold Remediation: Promptly address any signs of mold or water damage in the home by cleaning and removing mold-affected materials and fixing leaks or moisture issues.

By implementing these environmental adjustments, individuals with pneumonia and asthma can create a safer and healthier living environment that supports respiratory health and reduces the risk of exacerbations. It's essential to tailor environmental modifications to individual needs and preferences and consult with healthcare providers for personalized recommendations.

Stress Management Techniques for Managing Pneumonia and Asthma

Managing stress effectively is essential for individuals with pneumonia and asthma, as stress can exacerbate symptoms and weaken the immune system. By incorporating stress management techniques into daily routines, individuals can reduce stress levels, improve overall well-being, and better cope with the challenges of living with respiratory conditions. Here are some stress management techniques to consider:

1. **Deep Breathing Exercises**: Practice deep breathing techniques to promote relaxation and reduce stress. Try diaphragmatic breathing, also known as belly breathing, by inhaling deeply through the nose, expanding the abdomen, and exhaling slowly through the mouth. Repeat several times to calm the mind and body.

2. **Mindfulness Meditation**: Engage in mindfulness meditation practices to cultivate present moment awareness and develop a sense of calmness and inner peace. Focus on the sensations of the breath, body, or surroundings without judgment or attachment to thoughts.

3. **Progressive Muscle Relaxation**: Practice progressive muscle relaxation to release tension and promote physical and mental relaxation. Start by tensing and then gradually relaxing each muscle group in the body, starting from the toes and working up to the head.

4. **Yoga and Tai Chi**: Participate in gentle mind-body exercises such as yoga or tai chi to promote relaxation, improve flexibility, and reduce stress levels. These practices incorporate breathing techniques, gentle movements, and mindfulness to promote overall well-being.

5. **Exercise Regularly**: Engage in regular physical activity to reduce stress and improve mood. Choose activities that you enjoy, such as walking, swimming, cycling, or dancing, and aim for at least 30 minutes of moderate-intensity exercise most days of the week.

6. **Journaling**: Keep a stress journal to identify sources of stress, track emotions, and explore coping strategies. Write down thoughts, feelings, and experiences regularly to gain insight into stress triggers and develop healthier responses.

7. **Social Support**: Seek support from friends, family members, support groups, or mental health professionals to share experiences, express emotions, and receive encouragement and guidance. Building a support network can help alleviate stress and provide a sense of belonging and connection.

8. **Healthy Lifestyle Habits**: Maintain a healthy lifestyle by prioritizing adequate sleep, eating a balanced diet, limiting caffeine and alcohol intake, and avoiding tobacco use. These habits support overall well-being and resilience to stress.

9. **Time Management**: Organize tasks, prioritize responsibilities, and set realistic goals to reduce feelings of overwhelm and manage stress more effectively. Break tasks into smaller, manageable steps and delegate tasks when necessary.

10. **Mindful Relaxation Techniques**: Engage in activities that promote relaxation and enjoyment, such as listening to soothing music, practicing aromatherapy with essential oils, taking warm baths, or spending time in nature.

By incorporating these stress management techniques into daily routines, individuals with pneumonia and asthma can reduce stress levels, enhance coping abilities, and improve overall quality of life. It's essential to experiment with different techniques and find what works best for you, as everyone responds differently to stress management strategies. Additionally, don't hesitate to seek professional help if stress becomes overwhelming or impacts daily functioning.

Chapter 3

Herbal Remedies for Pneumonia and Asthma

Herbal remedies have been used for centuries to alleviate symptoms and support respiratory health in conditions such as pneumonia and asthma. While it's essential to consult with a healthcare professional before using herbal remedies, as they may interact with medications or exacerbate underlying conditions, many herbs have shown promise in providing relief from respiratory symptoms. Here are some herbal remedies commonly used for pneumonia and asthma:

1. **Eucalyptus**: Eucalyptus contains compounds called cineole, which have bronchodilator and anti-inflammatory properties. Eucalyptus oil can be used in steam inhalation or diluted in carrier oil for chest rubs to help relieve congestion and ease breathing.

2. **Ginger**: Ginger has anti-inflammatory and immune-boosting properties, making it beneficial for respiratory conditions. Ginger tea or ginger extracts can help soothe sore throat, reduce inflammation, and relieve asthma symptoms.

3. **Turmeric**: Curcumin, the active compound in turmeric, possesses anti-inflammatory and antioxidant properties that may help reduce inflammation in the airways and improve lung function. Turmeric can be consumed as a spice in cooking or taken as a supplement.

4. **Licorice Root**: Licorice root contains glycyrrhizin, which has expectorant and anti-inflammatory effects. Licorice root tea or extracts can help loosen mucus, soothe irritated airways, and reduce coughing associated with pneumonia and asthma.

5. **Ginseng**: Ginseng has adaptogenic properties that help the body adapt to stress and improve immune function. Siberian ginseng (Eleutherococcus senticosus) and American ginseng (Panax quinquefolius) may support respiratory health and enhance overall well-being.

6. **Peppermint**: Peppermint contains menthol, which has a cooling and soothing effect on the respiratory tract. Peppermint tea or peppermint oil in steam inhalation can help relieve congestion, open airways, and alleviate asthma symptoms.

7. **Thyme**: Thyme contains compounds like thymol and carvacrol, which have antimicrobial and expectorant properties. Thyme tea or thyme essential oil can help loosen mucus, relieve cough, and support respiratory health.

8. **Oregano**: Oregano contains carvacrol and rosmarinic acid, which have antimicrobial, anti-inflammatory, and bronchodilator properties. Oregano oil or oregano tea may help reduce inflammation, fight respiratory infections, and improve asthma symptoms.

9. **Garlic**: Garlic has antimicrobial, anti-inflammatory, and immune-boosting properties that may help support respiratory health. Consuming raw garlic or garlic supplements may help prevent respiratory infections and reduce asthma symptoms.

10. **Marshmallow Root**: Marshmallow root contains mucilage, a gel-like substance that coats and soothes the respiratory tract. Marshmallow root tea or extracts can help relieve cough, sore throat, and irritation associated with pneumonia and asthma.

While herbal remedies can provide symptomatic relief and support respiratory health, it's essential to use them cautiously and under the guidance of a healthcare professional. Some herbs may interact with medications or exacerbate underlying health conditions, and individual responses to herbal remedies can vary. Additionally, pregnant or breastfeeding individuals should exercise caution when using herbal remedies.

Eucalyptus for Pneumonia and Asthma

Eucalyptus is a popular herbal remedy known for its respiratory benefits, making it useful for managing symptoms of pneumonia and asthma. Here's how eucalyptus can be beneficial for these respiratory conditions:

1. **Bronchodilator Effect**: Eucalyptus contains a compound called cineole, which has bronchodilator properties. Bronchodilators help relax the muscles in the airways, making it easier to breathe. This effect can be particularly helpful for individuals with asthma who experience bronchoconstriction and airway constriction.

2. **Expectorant Properties**: Eucalyptus oil has expectorant properties, meaning it can help loosen and expel mucus from the respiratory tract. By thinning mucus and promoting its clearance, eucalyptus can alleviate congestion and facilitate easier breathing, which is beneficial for individuals with pneumonia and asthma.

3. **Anti-inflammatory Action**: The anti-inflammatory properties of eucalyptus oil can help reduce inflammation in the airways, making it effective for relieving symptoms such as coughing, wheezing, and chest tightness associated with pneumonia and asthma. By reducing airway inflammation, eucalyptus may help improve respiratory function and alleviate discomfort.

4. **Antimicrobial Effects**: Eucalyptus oil exhibits antimicrobial activity against bacteria, viruses, and fungi, which can help combat respiratory infections that may exacerbate pneumonia symptoms or trigger asthma attacks. Using eucalyptus oil in steam inhalation or diffusers may help kill or inhibit the growth of pathogens in the respiratory tract.

5. **Soothing Properties**: In addition to its respiratory benefits, eucalyptus oil has a cooling

and soothing effect on the throat and airways, providing relief from irritation and discomfort. This soothing action can help reduce coughing and throat irritation associated with pneumonia and asthma.

6. **Ease of Use**: Eucalyptus oil is easy to use and can be incorporated into various home remedies for respiratory relief. It can be diluted in carrier oils for chest rubs, added to hot water for steam inhalation, or used in aromatherapy diffusers to inhale its vapors.

It's important to note that while eucalyptus oil can provide symptomatic relief for pneumonia and asthma, it should be used with caution, especially in individuals with sensitive skin or respiratory conditions. Some people may be allergic to eucalyptus oil or experience irritation when inhaling its vapors. It's advisable to perform a patch test before using eucalyptus oil topically and to start with low concentrations when inhaling its vapors. Additionally, pregnant or breastfeeding individuals and children should consult with a healthcare professional before using eucalyptus oil.

Ginger for Pneumonia and Asthma

Ginger is a versatile herb with a long history of medicinal use, including for respiratory conditions like pneumonia and asthma. Here's how ginger can be beneficial for managing symptoms associated with these respiratory ailments:

1. **Anti-inflammatory Properties**: Ginger contains bioactive compounds like gingerol and shogaol, which exhibit potent anti-inflammatory effects. Inflammation in the airways is a common feature of both pneumonia and asthma. Consuming ginger may help reduce airway inflammation, easing symptoms such as coughing, chest tightness, and shortness of breath.

2. **Bronchodilator Effect**: Some studies suggest that ginger may have bronchodilator properties, meaning it can help relax the muscles in the airways and improve airflow. This bronchodilator effect may be beneficial for individuals with asthma, as it can help alleviate bronchoconstriction and ease breathing difficulties.

3. **Antimicrobial Activity**: Ginger possesses antimicrobial properties that may help combat respiratory infections caused by bacteria or viruses.

By inhibiting the growth of pathogens, ginger may help prevent or reduce the severity of pneumonia symptoms and support the body's immune response to infections.

4. **Expectorant Action**: Ginger has expectorant properties, which means it can help thin and expel mucus from the respiratory tract. By promoting mucus clearance, ginger may alleviate congestion, reduce coughing, and facilitate easier breathing for individuals with pneumonia or asthma.

5. **Immune-Boosting Effects**: The immune-boosting properties of ginger may help strengthen the body's defenses against respiratory infections and promote overall immune function. Consuming ginger regularly may help support respiratory health and reduce the risk of recurrent infections.

6. **Soothing Effect**: Ginger has a warming and soothing effect on the throat and respiratory tract, which can provide relief from irritation and discomfort associated with coughing, sore throat, and chest congestion. Ginger tea or throat lozenges made with ginger may help soothe respiratory symptoms and promote comfort.

7. **Ease of Use**: Ginger is easy to incorporate into the diet and can be consumed in various forms, including fresh ginger root, ginger tea, ginger supplements, or added to recipes. Drinking ginger tea or including ginger in meals may provide ongoing respiratory support and symptom relief.

While ginger can offer symptomatic relief for pneumonia and asthma, it's essential to use it as part of a comprehensive management plan and consult with a healthcare professional, especially if you have underlying health conditions or are taking medications. Additionally, individuals with gastroesophageal reflux disease (GERD) should use ginger with caution, as it may exacerbate reflux symptoms in some cases.

Turmeric for Pneumonia and Asthma

Turmeric, a golden-yellow spice commonly used in cooking and traditional medicine, offers several potential benefits for managing symptoms associated with pneumonia and asthma. Here's how turmeric can be beneficial:

1. **Anti-inflammatory Properties**: Curcumin, the active compound in turmeric, possesses potent

anti-inflammatory properties. Inflammation plays a key role in the pathogenesis of pneumonia and asthma, contributing to respiratory symptoms such as coughing, wheezing, and airway constriction. Consuming turmeric may help reduce inflammation in the airways, easing respiratory symptoms and promoting healing.

2. **Antioxidant Activity**: Curcumin is a powerful antioxidant that helps neutralize harmful free radicals in the body. Oxidative stress and damage contribute to inflammation and tissue injury in the lungs, exacerbating respiratory conditions like pneumonia and asthma. By scavenging free radicals, turmeric may protect against oxidative damage and support lung health.

3. **Immune Modulation**: Turmeric has immunomodulatory effects, meaning it can help regulate immune responses in the body. By modulating immune function, turmeric may help strengthen the immune system's ability to fight off infections, including those that cause pneumonia. Additionally, balanced immune function is essential for managing asthma and reducing the risk of exacerbations.

4. **Bronchodilator Activity**: Some studies suggest that turmeric may have bronchodilator properties, similar to conventional asthma medications. Bronchodilators help relax the muscles in the airways, improving airflow and easing breathing difficulties. Consuming turmeric may help alleviate bronchoconstriction and respiratory symptoms in individuals with asthma.

5. **Mucolytic Effects**: Turmeric has mucolytic properties, meaning it can help break down and expel excess mucus from the respiratory tract. Excessive mucus production and accumulation can exacerbate respiratory symptoms and hinder breathing. By promoting mucus clearance, turmeric may reduce congestion and facilitate easier breathing.

6. **Antimicrobial Activity**: Turmeric exhibits antimicrobial activity against bacteria, viruses, and fungi, which may help prevent or combat respiratory infections associated with pneumonia. Including turmeric in the diet or consuming turmeric supplements may support immune function and reduce the risk of infectious complications.

7. **Ease of Incorporation**: Turmeric is versatile and can be easily incorporated into various dishes, including curries, soups, stir-fries, and beverages like turmeric tea or golden milk. Adding turmeric to meals regularly may provide ongoing respiratory support and symptom relief.

While turmeric can offer potential benefits for managing pneumonia and asthma, it's essential to use it as part of a comprehensive treatment plan and consult with a healthcare professional, especially if you have underlying health conditions or are taking medications. Additionally, individuals with gallbladder disease or those at risk of kidney stones should use turmeric with caution, as it may exacerbate these conditions in some cases.

Licorice Root for Pneumonia and Asthma

Licorice root, derived from the Glycyrrhiza glabra plant, has been used for centuries in traditional medicine for its medicinal properties. When used appropriately, licorice root may offer several potential benefits for managing symptoms associated with pneumonia and asthma. Here's how licorice root can be beneficial:

1. **Expectorant Properties**: Licorice root contains compounds known as saponins, which have expectorant effects. Expectorants help loosen and expel mucus from the respiratory tract, making it easier to clear congestion and alleviate coughing associated with pneumonia and asthma.

2. **Anti-inflammatory Activity**: Licorice root contains glycyrrhizin, a compound with potent anti-inflammatory properties. Inflammation in the airways is a hallmark of respiratory conditions like pneumonia and asthma, contributing to symptoms such as coughing, wheezing, and chest tightness. Consuming licorice root may help reduce airway inflammation and alleviate respiratory symptoms.

3. **Soothing and Demulcent Effects**: Licorice root has demulcent properties, meaning it forms a soothing, protective coating over irritated mucous membranes in the throat and respiratory tract. This coating can help relieve sore throat, irritation, and cough associated with pneumonia and asthma, promoting comfort and symptom relief.

4. **Antiviral and Antimicrobial Effects**: Licorice root exhibits antiviral and antimicrobial activity against bacteria, viruses, and fungi. By inhibiting the growth of pathogens, licorice root

may help prevent respiratory infections that can exacerbate pneumonia symptoms or trigger asthma attacks.

5. **Bronchodilator Activity**: Some studies suggest that licorice root may have bronchodilator properties, helping to relax the muscles in the airways and improve airflow. This bronchodilator effect may be beneficial for individuals with asthma, as it can help alleviate bronchoconstriction and ease breathing difficulties.

6. **Immune Modulation**: Licorice root has immunomodulatory effects, meaning it can help regulate immune responses in the body. By modulating immune function, licorice root may support the body's ability to fight off respiratory infections and reduce the risk of complications associated with pneumonia and asthma.

7. **Ease of Use**: Licorice root can be consumed in various forms, including licorice tea, licorice supplements, or as a component of herbal formulations. Drinking licorice tea or taking licorice supplements may provide respiratory support and symptom relief.

It's important to note that licorice root should be used cautiously and under the guidance of a healthcare professional, as excessive consumption or prolonged use may lead to adverse effects, including elevated blood pressure, potassium depletion, and interactions with medications. Individuals with hypertension, heart disease, kidney disorders, or hormonal imbalances should avoid licorice root or use it under close supervision. Pregnant or breastfeeding individuals should also consult with a healthcare provider before using licorice root.

Ginseng for Pneumonia and Asthma

Ginseng, a well-known herbal remedy in traditional medicine, offers potential benefits for managing symptoms associated with pneumonia and asthma. Here's how ginseng can be beneficial:

1. **Adaptogenic Properties**: Ginseng is classified as an adaptogen, meaning it helps the body adapt to stress and maintain homeostasis. By supporting the body's ability to cope with physical and environmental stressors, ginseng may help reduce the severity of pneumonia symptoms and asthma exacerbations triggered by stress.

2. **Immune Modulation**: Ginseng has immunomodulatory effects, meaning it can regulate immune responses in the body. By modulating immune function, ginseng may help strengthen the immune system's ability to fight off respiratory infections and reduce the risk of complications associated with pneumonia and asthma.

3. **Anti-inflammatory Activity**: Ginseng contains bioactive compounds such as ginsenosides, which have anti-inflammatory properties. Inflammation in the airways contributes to respiratory symptoms such as coughing, wheezing, and chest tightness. Consuming ginseng may help reduce airway inflammation and alleviate respiratory symptoms.

4. **Bronchodilator Effects**: Some studies suggest that ginseng may have bronchodilator properties, similar to conventional asthma medications. Bronchodilators help relax the muscles in the airways, improving airflow and easing breathing difficulties. Consuming ginseng may help alleviate bronchoconstriction and respiratory symptoms in individuals with asthma.

5. **Antioxidant Activity**: Ginseng exhibits antioxidant properties, helping to neutralize

harmful free radicals in the body. Oxidative stress and damage contribute to inflammation and tissue injury in the lungs, exacerbating respiratory conditions like pneumonia and asthma. By scavenging free radicals, ginseng may protect against oxidative damage and support lung health.

6. **Energy and Vitality**: Ginseng is known for its ability to enhance energy levels and improve overall vitality. Individuals recovering from pneumonia or managing asthma may benefit from ginseng's energizing effects, which can help combat fatigue and promote physical resilience.

7. **Stress Reduction**: Ginseng may help reduce stress and anxiety, which can exacerbate symptoms of pneumonia and asthma. By promoting relaxation and mental well-being, ginseng may support overall respiratory health and enhance coping abilities during times of illness or respiratory distress.

Ginseng is available in various forms, including ginseng tea, ginseng supplements, and herbal formulations. It's important to choose high-quality ginseng products from reputable sources and follow recommended dosages. Additionally, individuals with certain medical conditions or taking medications should consult with a healthcare professional before using ginseng to ensure safety and efficacy.

Chapter 4

Essential Oils for Respiratory Health

Essential oils are concentrated plant extracts that contain aromatic compounds with various therapeutic properties. When used safely and appropriately, certain essential oils can provide respiratory support and help alleviate symptoms associated with conditions like pneumonia and asthma. Here are some essential oils known for their respiratory benefits:

1. **Eucalyptus Oil**: Eucalyptus oil is well-known for its decongestant, expectorant, and bronchodilator properties. Inhalation of eucalyptus oil vapor can help clear nasal congestion, loosen mucus, and improve airflow in the respiratory tract. It's commonly used in steam inhalation, diffusers, or chest rubs for respiratory relief.

2. **Peppermint Oil**: Peppermint oil contains menthol, which has a cooling and soothing effect on the respiratory tract. Inhalation of peppermint oil vapor can help relieve nasal congestion, reduce coughing, and ease breathing difficulties. Peppermint oil can be used in steam inhalation, diffusers, or diluted in carrier oils for chest rubs.

3. **Tea Tree Oil**: Tea tree oil possesses antimicrobial and anti-inflammatory properties, making it useful for combating respiratory infections and reducing inflammation in the airways. Inhalation of tea tree oil vapor may help alleviate symptoms such as coughing, throat irritation, and congestion. It can be used in diffusers or steam inhalation.

4. **Lavender Oil**: Lavender oil is known for its calming and soothing properties, which can help reduce stress and promote relaxation. Inhalation of lavender oil vapor may help ease respiratory symptoms exacerbated by stress or anxiety. Lavender oil can be used in diffusers or added to bathwater for inhalation.

5. **Rosemary Oil**: Rosemary oil has expectorant and bronchodilator effects, making it beneficial for respiratory conditions like asthma and bronchitis. Inhalation of rosemary oil vapor can help loosen mucus, improve airflow, and relieve coughing. It can be used in steam inhalation or diffusers.

6. **Thyme Oil**: Thyme oil contains thymol, a compound with antimicrobial and expectorant properties. Inhalation of thyme oil vapor can help combat respiratory infections, loosen mucus, and

alleviate coughing. Thyme oil can be used in steam inhalation or diffusers.

7. **Frankincense Oil**: Frankincense oil has anti-inflammatory and immune-stimulating properties, which may help support respiratory health and reduce inflammation in the airways. Inhalation of frankincense oil vapor may help alleviate symptoms such as coughing and chest tightness. It can be used in diffusers or diluted in carrier oils for chest rubs.

8. **Lemon Oil**: Lemon oil contains limonene, a compound with decongestant and immune-boosting properties. Inhalation of lemon oil vapor can help clear nasal congestion, support immune function, and promote respiratory health. Lemon oil can be used in diffusers or added to steam inhalation.

When using essential oils for respiratory health, it's essential to follow safety guidelines and use them appropriately. Always dilute essential oils in carrier oils before applying them to the skin, and perform a patch test to check for sensitivity. Inhalation of essential oil vapor should be done in moderation to avoid irritation, and individuals with respiratory conditions should consult with a healthcare professional before using essential oils, especially if they have asthma or other respiratory sensitivities.

Peppermint Oil for Respiratory Health

Peppermint oil is renowned for its refreshing aroma and numerous therapeutic properties, including benefits for respiratory health. Here's how peppermint oil can be advantageous:

1. **Decongestant Effect**: Peppermint oil contains menthol, a compound known for its ability to act as a natural decongestant. Inhaling peppermint oil vapor can help clear nasal passages, reduce congestion, and alleviate respiratory symptoms associated with conditions like pneumonia and asthma.

2. **Bronchodilator Properties**: Menthol in peppermint oil also acts as a bronchodilator, helping to relax the muscles in the airways and improve airflow. This bronchodilator effect can be beneficial for individuals with asthma, as it may help alleviate bronchoconstriction and ease breathing difficulties.

3. **Expectorant Action**: Peppermint oil has expectorant properties, meaning it can help thin and loosen mucus in the respiratory tract, making it easier to expel. By promoting mucus clearance, peppermint oil may alleviate congestion, reduce coughing, and facilitate easier breathing.

4. **Anti-inflammatory Effects**: Peppermint oil exhibits anti-inflammatory properties, which can help reduce inflammation in the airways and alleviate respiratory symptoms such as coughing, wheezing, and chest tightness. By calming inflammation, peppermint oil may promote respiratory comfort and support lung health.

5. **Antimicrobial Activity**: Peppermint oil possesses antimicrobial properties that can help combat respiratory infections caused by bacteria, viruses, or fungi. Inhaling peppermint oil vapor may help reduce the risk of respiratory infections and support the body's immune response to infections.

6. **Soothing and Cooling Sensation**: The cooling sensation of peppermint oil can provide immediate relief from throat irritation, coughing, and discomfort associated with respiratory conditions. Inhaling peppermint oil vapor or

applying diluted oil to the chest can soothe the respiratory tract and promote comfort.

7. **Stress Reduction**: Peppermint oil's invigorating aroma can help reduce stress and promote relaxation, which is beneficial for individuals managing respiratory conditions exacerbated by stress or anxiety. Inhaling peppermint oil vapor can help calm the mind and enhance overall well-being.

Peppermint oil can be used in various ways to support respiratory health, including:

- **Steam Inhalation**: Add a few drops of peppermint oil to hot water and inhale the steam to clear nasal passages and relieve congestion.
- **Diffusion**: Use a diffuser to disperse peppermint oil vapor into the air, creating a refreshing and invigorating atmosphere that supports respiratory comfort.
- **Topical Application**: Dilute peppermint oil in a carrier oil (such as coconut or jojoba oil) and apply it to the chest or throat for soothing relief from respiratory symptoms.
- **Aromatherapy**: Add a few drops of peppermint oil to a warm bath or shower to enjoy its aromatic benefits and promote relaxation.

It's essential to use peppermint oil safely and appropriately, as concentrated essential oils can be potent and may cause skin irritation or allergic reactions in some individuals. Always dilute peppermint oil before applying it to the skin, and perform a patch test to check for sensitivity. If you have asthma or other respiratory conditions, consult with a healthcare professional before using peppermint oil to ensure compatibility and safety.

Tea Tree Oil for Respiratory Health

Tea tree oil, derived from the leaves of the Melaleuca alternifolia tree, is renowned for its antimicrobial and anti-inflammatory properties. While it is commonly associated with skin care, tea tree oil also offers benefits for respiratory health. Here's how tea tree oil can support respiratory wellness:

1. **Antimicrobial Activity**: Tea tree oil exhibits potent antimicrobial properties, making it effective against bacteria, viruses, and fungi. Inhaling tea tree oil vapor or using it in a diffuser can help purify the air and reduce the risk of respiratory infections that may exacerbate conditions like pneumonia or asthma.

2. **Decongestant Effect**: Tea tree oil has natural decongestant properties, which can help clear nasal passages and alleviate congestion in the respiratory tract. Inhaling tea tree oil vapor can provide relief from nasal congestion, sinus pressure, and respiratory discomfort associated with respiratory illnesses.

3. **Anti-inflammatory Action**: Tea tree oil possesses anti-inflammatory properties that can help reduce inflammation in the airways and ease respiratory symptoms such as coughing, wheezing, and chest tightness. Inhaling tea tree oil vapor may help calm inflammation and promote respiratory comfort.

4. **Expectorant Properties**: Tea tree oil has expectorant effects, meaning it can help loosen and expel mucus from the respiratory tract. By promoting mucus clearance, tea tree oil may alleviate congestion, reduce coughing, and facilitate easier breathing for individuals with pneumonia or asthma.

5. **Immune Support**: Tea tree oil can help support the immune system's ability to defend against respiratory infections. Inhaling tea tree oil vapor or using it in a diffuser may stimulate the

body's natural defenses and reduce the likelihood of respiratory illnesses.

6. **Stress Reduction**: The invigorating aroma of tea tree oil can help reduce stress and promote relaxation, which is beneficial for individuals managing respiratory conditions exacerbated by stress or anxiety. Inhaling tea tree oil vapor can help calm the mind and enhance overall well-being.

Tea tree oil can be used in various ways to support respiratory health, including:

- **Steam Inhalation**: Add a few drops of tea tree oil to hot water and inhale the steam to clear nasal passages, relieve congestion, and promote respiratory comfort.
- **Diffusion**: Use a diffuser to disperse tea tree oil vapor into the air, creating a clean and refreshing atmosphere that supports respiratory wellness.
- **Topical Application**: Dilute tea tree oil in a carrier oil (such as coconut or almond oil) and apply it to the chest or throat for soothing relief from respiratory symptoms.
- **Aromatherapy**: Add a few drops of tea tree oil to a warm bath or shower to enjoy its aromatic benefits and promote relaxation.

It's important to use tea tree oil safely and appropriately, as concentrated essential oils can be potent and may cause skin irritation or allergic reactions in some individuals. Always dilute tea tree oil before applying it to the skin, and perform a patch test to check for sensitivity. If you have asthma or other respiratory conditions, consult with a healthcare professional before using tea tree oil to ensure compatibility and safety.

Lavender Oil for Respiratory Health

Lavender oil, derived from the lavender plant (Lavandula angustifolia), is well-known for its calming aroma and numerous therapeutic properties. While it is often associated with relaxation and stress relief, lavender oil also offers benefits for respiratory health. Here's how lavender oil can support respiratory wellness:

1. **Relaxation and Stress Reduction**: Lavender oil is renowned for its calming and soothing effects on the mind and body. Inhaling lavender oil vapor or using it in aromatherapy can help reduce stress and anxiety, which are common triggers for respiratory symptoms. By promoting relaxation,

lavender oil may indirectly support respiratory health and improve overall well-being.

2. **Anti-inflammatory Properties**: Lavender oil possesses anti-inflammatory properties that can help reduce inflammation in the airways and alleviate respiratory symptoms such as coughing, wheezing, and chest tightness. Inhaling lavender oil vapor may help calm inflammation and promote respiratory comfort.

3. **Antimicrobial Activity**: Lavender oil exhibits antimicrobial properties, making it effective against bacteria, viruses, and fungi. Inhaling lavender oil vapor or using it in a diffuser can help purify the air and reduce the risk of respiratory infections that may exacerbate conditions like pneumonia or asthma.

4. **Decongestant Effect**: Lavender oil has mild decongestant properties, which can help clear nasal passages and alleviate congestion in the respiratory tract. Inhaling lavender oil vapor can provide relief from nasal congestion, sinus pressure, and respiratory discomfort associated with respiratory illnesses.

5. **Sleep Support**: Lavender oil is often used to promote relaxation and improve sleep quality. Adequate sleep is essential for maintaining respiratory health and supporting immune function. Using lavender oil in aromatherapy before bedtime may help promote restful sleep and enhance overall respiratory wellness.

6. **Mood Enhancement**: The pleasant aroma of lavender oil can uplift the mood and promote a sense of well-being. Inhaling lavender oil vapor can help improve mood and reduce feelings of anxiety or depression, which may positively impact respiratory health.

Lavender oil can be used in various ways to support respiratory health, including:

- **Diffusion**: Use a diffuser to disperse lavender oil vapor into the air, creating a calming and relaxing atmosphere that promotes respiratory comfort.
- **Aromatherapy**: Add a few drops of lavender oil to a warm bath or shower to enjoy its aromatic benefits and promote relaxation before bedtime.
- **Topical Application**: Dilute lavender oil in a carrier oil (such as coconut or almond oil) and apply it to the chest or throat for soothing relief from respiratory symptoms.

It's important to use lavender oil safely and appropriately, as concentrated essential oils can be potent and may cause skin irritation or allergic reactions in some individuals. Always dilute lavender oil before applying it to the skin, and perform a patch test to check for sensitivity. If you have asthma or other respiratory conditions, consult with a healthcare professional before using lavender oil to ensure compatibility and safety.

Eucalyptus Oil for Respiratory Health

Eucalyptus oil, extracted from the leaves of the eucalyptus tree (Eucalyptus globulus), is renowned for its refreshing aroma and numerous therapeutic properties, particularly for respiratory health. Here's how eucalyptus oil can support respiratory wellness:

1. **Decongestant Effect**: Eucalyptus oil contains a compound called cineole, which has natural decongestant properties. Inhaling eucalyptus oil vapor can help clear nasal passages, reduce sinus congestion, and alleviate respiratory symptoms such as coughing and wheezing.

2. **Expectorant Properties**: Eucalyptus oil has expectorant effects, meaning it can help loosen and expel mucus from the respiratory tract. By promoting mucus clearance, eucalyptus oil may alleviate congestion, reduce coughing, and facilitate easier breathing for individuals with respiratory conditions like pneumonia or asthma.

3. **Bronchodilator Action**: Cineole in eucalyptus oil also acts as a bronchodilator, helping to relax the muscles in the airways and improve airflow. This bronchodilator effect can be beneficial for individuals with asthma, as it may help alleviate bronchoconstriction and ease breathing difficulties.

4. **Anti-inflammatory Properties**: Eucalyptus oil possesses anti-inflammatory properties that can help reduce inflammation in the airways and alleviate respiratory symptoms such as coughing, wheezing, and chest tightness. Inhaling eucalyptus oil vapor may help calm inflammation and promote respiratory comfort.

5. **Antimicrobial Activity**: Eucalyptus oil exhibits antimicrobial properties, making it effective against bacteria, viruses, and fungi. Inhaling eucalyptus oil vapor or using it in a diffuser can help purify the air and reduce the risk of respiratory infections that

may exacerbate conditions like pneumonia or asthma.

6. **Sinus Relief**: Eucalyptus oil's refreshing aroma can provide immediate relief from sinus pressure and congestion. Inhaling eucalyptus oil vapor or using it in steam inhalation can help clear nasal passages and promote sinus drainage, relieving discomfort associated with sinusitis or allergies.

7. **Mood Enhancement**: The invigorating scent of eucalyptus oil can uplift the mood and promote a sense of clarity and well-being. Inhaling eucalyptus oil vapor can help improve focus and mental alertness, which may positively impact respiratory health.

Eucalyptus oil can be used in various ways to support respiratory health, including:

- **Steam Inhalation**: Add a few drops of eucalyptus oil to hot water and inhale the steam to clear nasal passages, relieve congestion, and promote respiratory comfort.
- **Diffusion**: Use a diffuser to disperse eucalyptus oil vapor into the air, creating a refreshing and invigorating atmosphere that supports respiratory wellness.

- **Topical Application**: Dilute eucalyptus oil in a carrier oil (such as coconut or almond oil) and apply it to the chest or throat for soothing relief from respiratory symptoms.

It's important to use eucalyptus oil safely and appropriately, as concentrated essential oils can be potent and may cause skin irritation or allergic reactions in some individuals. Always dilute eucalyptus oil before applying it to the skin, and perform a patch test to check for sensitivity. If you have asthma or other respiratory conditions, consult with a healthcare professional before using eucalyptus oil to ensure compatibility and safety.

Oregano Oil for Respiratory Health

Oregano oil, derived from the leaves of the oregano plant (Origanum vulgare), is a potent herbal remedy known for its antimicrobial and anti-inflammatory properties. While it is commonly used for culinary purposes, oregano oil also offers benefits for respiratory health. Here's how oregano oil can support respiratory wellness:

1. **Antimicrobial Activity**: Oregano oil contains compounds such as carvacrol and thymol, which

have strong antimicrobial properties. Inhaling oregano oil vapor or using it in a diffuser can help purify the air and reduce the risk of respiratory infections caused by bacteria, viruses, or fungi.

2. **Immune Support**: Oregano oil can help support the immune system's ability to defend against respiratory infections. Inhaling oregano oil vapor or using it in aromatherapy may stimulate the body's natural defenses and reduce the likelihood of respiratory illnesses.

3. **Anti-inflammatory Properties**: Oregano oil possesses anti-inflammatory properties that can help reduce inflammation in the airways and alleviate respiratory symptoms such as coughing, wheezing, and chest tightness. Inhaling oregano oil vapor may help calm inflammation and promote respiratory comfort.

4. **Expectorant Effects**: Oregano oil has expectorant properties, meaning it can help loosen and expel mucus from the respiratory tract. By promoting mucus clearance, oregano oil may alleviate congestion, reduce coughing, and facilitate easier breathing for individuals with respiratory conditions like pneumonia or asthma.

5. **Antioxidant Activity**: Oregano oil is rich in antioxidants, which help neutralize harmful free radicals in the body. Oxidative stress and damage contribute to inflammation and tissue injury in the lungs, exacerbating respiratory conditions like pneumonia and asthma. By scavenging free radicals, oregano oil may protect against oxidative damage and support lung health.

6. **Sinus Relief**: Oregano oil's aromatic properties can provide relief from sinus congestion and pressure. Inhaling oregano oil vapor or using it in steam inhalation can help clear nasal passages and promote sinus drainage, relieving discomfort associated with sinusitis or allergies.

7. **Mood Enhancement**: The invigorating scent of oregano oil can uplift the mood and promote a sense of well-being. Inhaling oregano oil vapor can help improve mood and reduce feelings of anxiety or stress, which may positively impact respiratory health.

Oregano oil can be used in various ways to support respiratory health, including:

- **Steam Inhalation**: Add a few drops of oregano oil to hot water and inhale the steam to clear nasal

passages, relieve congestion, and promote respiratory comfort.
- **Diffusion**: Use a diffuser to disperse oregano oil vapor into the air, creating a clean and refreshing atmosphere that supports respiratory wellness.
- **Topical Application**: Dilute oregano oil in a carrier oil (such as coconut or olive oil) and apply it to the chest or throat for soothing relief from respiratory symptoms.

It's important to use oregano oil safely and appropriately, as concentrated essential oils can be potent and may cause skin irritation or allergic reactions in some individuals. Always dilute oregano oil before applying it to the skin, and perform a patch test to check for sensitivity. If you have asthma or other respiratory conditions, consult with a healthcare professional before using oregano oil to ensure compatibility and safety.

Chapter 5

Homeopathic Remedies for Pneumonia and Asthma

Homeopathy offers a holistic approach to treating various health conditions, including pneumonia and asthma. Homeopathic remedies are derived from natural substances and are selected based on the principle of "like cures like" and individualized symptom patterns. While homeopathy should be used under the guidance of a qualified homeopathic practitioner, here are some commonly used remedies for pneumonia and asthma:

Homeopathic Remedies for Pneumonia:

1. **Antimonium Tartaricum (Ant-t.):** Used for pneumonia with rattling mucus, difficulty breathing, and a feeling of suffocation. The person may have a wet cough that produces thick, yellow-green mucus.

2. **Bryonia Alba (Bry.):** Indicated for pneumonia with dry, painful cough that worsens with movement or deep breathing. The person may

experience stitching pains in the chest and prefer to lie still.

3. Hepar Sulphuris Calcareum (Hep.): Helpful for pneumonia with sharp, splinter-like pains in the chest and a loose, rattling cough. The cough may be worse at night and accompanied by yellow or green sputum.

4. Phosphorus (Phos.): Used for pneumonia with weakness, fever, and a dry, tickling cough. The person may have a burning sensation in the chest and cough up bright red or bloody sputum.

5. Arsenicum Album (Ars.): Indicated for pneumonia with intense anxiety, restlessness, and a dry, burning cough. The person may feel worse at night and have difficulty breathing, especially when lying down.

Homeopathic Remedies for Asthma:

1. Arsenicum Album (Ars.): Used for asthma with anxiety, restlessness, and difficulty breathing. The person may experience wheezing, coughing, and a sense of suffocation, worsened by cold air and exertion.

2. **Natrum Sulphuricum (Nat-s.)**: Indicated for asthma triggered by dampness or changes in weather. The person may experience wheezing, coughing, and difficulty breathing, particularly in the morning or after exertion.

3. **Sambucus Nigra (Samb.)**: Helpful for asthma with sudden onset of breathlessness, especially at night. The person may wake up feeling suffocated, with difficulty exhaling.

4. **Ipecacuanha (Ip.)**: Used for asthma with persistent coughing, wheezing, and difficulty breathing. The person may experience nausea and vomiting, with a sensation of constriction in the chest.

5. **Spongia Tosta (Spong.)**: Indicated for asthma with dry, barking cough, wheezing, and difficulty breathing, especially at night. The person may feel as if the throat is dry and constricted.

It's important to consult with a qualified homeopathic practitioner for proper diagnosis and individualized treatment. Homeopathic remedies should be selected based on the unique symptoms and characteristics of each individual, and treatment may involve a combination of remedies tailored to the person's specific needs. Additionally, homeopathic treatment should be used alongside conventional medical care for conditions like pneumonia and asthma.

Antimonium Tartaricum (Ant-t.)

Antimonium Tartaricum, also known as Tartar Emetic, is a homeopathic remedy derived from potassium antimony tartrate. It is commonly used to address respiratory conditions characterized by rattling mucus, difficulty breathing, and a feeling of suffocation, making it particularly suitable for pneumonia. Here's how Antimonium Tartaricum may be beneficial:

1. **Rattling Mucus**: Antimonium Tartaricum is indicated when the lungs are filled with excessive mucus, causing a rattling sound during breathing. This remedy helps to loosen and expectorate thick, tenacious mucus, promoting easier breathing and aiding in the resolution of pneumonia symptoms.

2. **Difficulty Breathing**: Individuals who require Antimonium Tartaricum often experience labored breathing, with a sensation of heaviness and oppression in the chest. They may feel as if they

cannot get enough air and may exhibit shallow, rapid breathing.

3. **Cough**: The cough associated with Antimonium Tartaricum pneumonia is typically loose and productive, with the inability to expectorate the mucus effectively. The cough may be accompanied by wheezing and chest congestion.

4. **Drowsiness and Weakness**: Individuals in need of Antimonium Tartaricum may feel weak, drowsy, and apathetic. They may prefer to lie down and may exhibit a lack of energy or desire to move.

5. **Coldness**: Despite the presence of fever or inflammation, individuals requiring Antimonium Tartaricum may feel chilly and desire warmth. They may have cold, clammy skin and a general aversion to cold air or drafts.

6. **Thirstlessness**: Unlike some other homeopathic remedies for pneumonia, individuals needing Antimonium Tartaricum may not exhibit excessive thirst. They may have little desire to drink fluids, even when experiencing fever or dehydration.

Antimonium Tartaricum is typically administered in low potencies, such as 6C or 30C, depending on the severity and individual response to treatment. As with all homeopathic remedies, it's important to consult with a qualified homeopathic practitioner for proper diagnosis and personalized treatment. While Antimonium Tartaricum can be a valuable remedy for pneumonia, it should be used as part of a comprehensive treatment plan, which may include conventional medical interventions as needed.

Arsenicum Album (Ars.)

Arsenicum Album, also known as Arsenic trioxide, is a widely used homeopathic remedy derived from arsenic. It is commonly prescribed for a range of conditions, including respiratory ailments like asthma, especially when symptoms are characterized by anxiety, restlessness, and difficulty breathing. Here's how Arsenicum Album may be beneficial for asthma:

1. **Anxiety and Restlessness**: Arsenicum Album is indicated when there is intense anxiety and restlessness, particularly during asthma attacks.

Individuals may feel agitated, fearful, and may seek constant reassurance from others.

2. **Difficulty Breathing**: This remedy is particularly useful for asthma attacks characterized by difficulty breathing, wheezing, and shortness of breath. Breathing may be rapid, shallow, and labored, with a sensation of suffocation or constriction in the chest.

3. **Burning Sensation**: Arsenicum Album is known for its affinity for conditions with burning pains, and individuals may experience a burning sensation in the chest during asthma attacks. The throat may also feel dry and constricted, exacerbating breathing difficulties.

4. **Worsening at Night**: Asthma symptoms requiring Arsenicum Album are often worse at night, disrupting sleep and causing anxiety. Individuals may wake up feeling suffocated and may experience an exacerbation of symptoms in the early hours of the morning.

5. **Thirst for Small Sips of Water**: Despite the burning sensations and dryness, individuals needing Arsenicum Album may crave small sips of water. They may be anxious about becoming

dehydrated and may have a compulsive need to drink frequently.

6. **Weakness and Exhaustion**: Following an asthma attack, individuals may feel weak, exhausted, and debilitated. Arsenicum Album helps to address these feelings of weakness and promotes recovery after the acute phase of the attack.

7. **Aggravation from Cold Air**: Asthma symptoms may be aggravated by exposure to cold air or drafts. Individuals requiring Arsenicum Album may feel worse in cold, damp environments and may seek warmth and comfort.

Arsenicum Album is typically administered in low potencies, such as 6C or 30C, depending on the severity and individual response to treatment. As with all homeopathic remedies, it's important to consult with a qualified homeopathic practitioner for proper diagnosis and personalized treatment. While Arsenicum Album can be a valuable remedy for asthma, it should be used as part of a comprehensive treatment plan, which may include conventional medical interventions as needed.

Bryonia Alba (Bry.)

Bryonia Alba, also known as Wild Hops or White Bryony, is a homeopathic remedy derived from the root of the Bryonia plant. It is commonly used to address respiratory conditions like pneumonia and asthma, particularly when symptoms are characterized by dryness, stitching pains, and aggravation from movement. Here's how Bryonia may be beneficial for respiratory health:

1. **Dry Cough**: Bryonia is indicated for respiratory conditions with a dry, hacking cough that is aggravated by movement, talking, or deep breathing. The cough may be painful and may cause soreness in the chest or abdomen.

2. **Stitching Chest Pains**: Individuals requiring Bryonia often experience sharp, stitching pains in the chest, worsened by coughing or deep inspiration. The chest may feel tight and sore, as if it is being constricted.

3. **Fever with Thirst**: Bryonia is often prescribed for individuals with fever, particularly if they experience intense thirst for large quantities of cold water. Despite the fever, individuals may have dry

mucous membranes and may be averse to warm drinks.

4. **Aggravation from Movement**: Symptoms of pneumonia or asthma requiring Bryonia are typically aggravated by any form of movement. Individuals may prefer to lie still and may be reluctant to change position due to the exacerbation of symptoms.

5. **Dryness of Mucous Membranes**: Bryonia is associated with dryness of mucous membranes throughout the body, including the respiratory tract. Individuals may complain of dryness and irritation in the throat, with little expectoration of mucus.

6. **Irritability and Grumpiness**: Individuals needing Bryonia may exhibit irritability and a desire to be left alone. They may become easily annoyed or angered, particularly when their symptoms are aggravated.

7. **Slow Onset of Symptoms**: Symptoms of pneumonia or asthma requiring Bryonia often develop gradually over time, with a slow onset of fever, cough, and chest pain. The individual may

initially attempt to suppress symptoms but eventually seek relief as the condition worsens.

Bryonia is typically administered in low to medium potencies, such as 6C or 30C, depending on the severity and individual response to treatment. As with all homeopathic remedies, it's important to consult with a qualified homeopathic practitioner for proper diagnosis and personalized treatment. While Bryonia can be a valuable remedy for respiratory conditions, it should be used as part of a comprehensive treatment plan, which may include conventional medical interventions as needed.

Ipecacuanha (Ip.)

Ipecacuanha, commonly known as Ipecac, is a homeopathic remedy derived from the root of the Ipecacuanha plant. It is frequently used to address respiratory conditions such as asthma, particularly when symptoms are characterized by persistent coughing, wheezing, and difficulty breathing. Here's how Ipecacuanha may be beneficial for respiratory health:

1. **Persistent Coughing**: Ipecacuanha is indicated for individuals with asthma who experience

relentless, spasmodic coughing that is difficult to suppress. The cough may be dry and suffocative, with a sensation of constriction or tightness in the chest.

2. **Wheezing**: Individuals requiring Ipecacuanha often exhibit wheezing, particularly during asthma attacks. The wheezing may be loud and raspy, accompanied by a sensation of tightness or constriction in the chest.

3. **Difficulty Breathing**: Ipecacuanha is useful for asthma attacks characterized by difficulty breathing, shortness of breath, and a feeling of suffocation. Breathing may be rapid, shallow, and labored, with a sense of heaviness in the chest.

4. **Nausea and Vomiting**: In addition to respiratory symptoms, individuals requiring Ipecacuanha may experience nausea and vomiting, particularly during asthma attacks. There may be a persistent sensation of nausea, with a tendency to vomit mucus or phlegm.

5. **Clean Tongue**: Unlike some other homeopathic remedies for respiratory conditions, individuals needing Ipecacuanha typically have a clean tongue without coating or discoloration. This

characteristic, along with the presence of nausea, helps differentiate it from other remedies.

6. **Suffocative Attacks**: Ipecacuanha is particularly useful for asthma attacks that feel suffocative, with a sense of tightness or constriction in the chest that makes breathing difficult. The individual may feel as if they cannot get enough air and may panic during the attack.

7. **Aggravation from Motion**: Symptoms of asthma requiring Ipecacuanha are often aggravated by any form of motion or exertion. The individual may prefer to lie still and may become agitated or anxious if forced to move.

Ipecacuanha is typically administered in low to medium potencies, such as 6C or 30C, depending on the severity and individual response to treatment. As with all homeopathic remedies, it's important to consult with a qualified homeopathic practitioner for proper diagnosis and personalized treatment. While Ipecacuanha can be a valuable remedy for asthma, it should be used as part of a comprehensive treatment plan, which may include conventional medical interventions as needed.

Spongia Tosta (Spong.)

Spongia Tosta, derived from roasted sponge, is a homeopathic remedy commonly used to address respiratory conditions, particularly asthma. It is indicated when symptoms include dry, barking cough, wheezing, and difficulty breathing, especially at night. Here's how Spongia Tosta may be beneficial for respiratory health:

1. **Dry, Barking Cough**: Spongia Tosta is well-suited for individuals with a dry, barking cough resembling the sound of a saw or a seal. The cough may be harsh, rasping, and repetitive, with a tendency to occur in paroxysms.

2. **Wheezing**: Individuals requiring Spongia Tosta often exhibit wheezing, particularly during asthma attacks. The wheezing may be loud, coarse, and croupy, resembling the sound of a saw or a whistle.

3. **Difficulty Breathing**: Spongia Tosta is indicated for asthma attacks characterized by difficulty breathing, shortness of breath, and a sense of constriction or tightness in the chest. Breathing may be labored, with a sensation of suffocation or oppression.

4. **Aggravation at Night**: Symptoms of asthma requiring Spongia Tosta are typically worse at night, particularly around midnight or in the early hours of the morning. The individual may wake up feeling suffocated and may experience an exacerbation of symptoms upon lying down.

5. **Throat Dryness**: Individuals needing Spongia Tosta may complain of dryness and irritation in the throat, with a sensation of rawness or scratching. The throat may feel dry and parched, exacerbating coughing and breathing difficulties.

6. **Relief from Warmth**: Spongia Tosta symptoms are often ameliorated by warmth and aggravated by cold air or drafts. The individual may seek warmth and comfort, preferring to be in a warm room or wrapped in blankets.

7. **Restlessness and Anxiety**: During asthma attacks, individuals requiring Spongia Tosta may experience restlessness and anxiety, particularly when breathing becomes difficult. They may feel apprehensive about the sensation of suffocation and may seek reassurance from others.

Spongia Tosta is typically administered in low to medium potencies, such as 6C or 30C, depending on the severity and individual response to treatment. As with all homeopathic remedies, it's important to consult with a qualified homeopathic practitioner for proper diagnosis and personalized treatment. While Spongia Tosta can be a valuable remedy for asthma, it should be used as part of a comprehensive treatment plan, which may include conventional medical interventions as needed.

Chapter 6

Dietary Supplements for Respiratory Support

Dietary supplements can play a supportive role in promoting respiratory health by providing essential nutrients and antioxidants that support lung function and immune response. Here are some dietary supplements that may be beneficial for respiratory support:

1. **Vitamin C**: Vitamin C is a powerful antioxidant that helps protect the respiratory tract from oxidative stress and inflammation. It also supports immune function and may reduce the severity and duration of respiratory infections.

2. **Vitamin D**: Vitamin D plays a crucial role in immune regulation and may help reduce the risk of respiratory infections. Adequate vitamin D levels have been associated with improved lung function and decreased susceptibility to respiratory illnesses.

3. **Omega-3 Fatty Acids**: Omega-3 fatty acids, found in fish oil and flaxseed oil, have anti-inflammatory properties that may help reduce

airway inflammation and improve lung function in individuals with respiratory conditions like asthma and COPD.

4. **Magnesium**: Magnesium is involved in muscle relaxation and may help alleviate bronchospasm and improve respiratory function in individuals with asthma. It also supports overall muscle and nerve function.

5. **N-acetylcysteine (NAC)**: NAC is a precursor to glutathione, a potent antioxidant that plays a key role in protecting lung tissue from damage. NAC supplementation may help reduce mucus viscosity and improve cough clearance in individuals with respiratory conditions.

6. **Quercetin**: Quercetin is a flavonoid with anti-inflammatory and antioxidant properties that may help reduce airway inflammation and improve lung function. It also supports immune function and may help prevent respiratory infections.

7. **Probiotics**: Probiotics are beneficial bacteria that support gut health and immune function. They may help reduce the risk of respiratory infections by modulating the immune response and promoting a healthy balance of gut microbiota.

8. **Zinc**: Zinc is essential for immune function and may help reduce the severity and duration of respiratory infections. It also plays a role in wound healing and may support respiratory tissue repair.

9. **Selenium**: Selenium is an antioxidant mineral that helps protect lung tissue from oxidative damage. Adequate selenium levels have been associated with improved lung function and reduced risk of respiratory infections.

10. **Elderberry**: Elderberry is rich in antioxidants and has antiviral properties that may help reduce the severity and duration of colds and flu. It may also help alleviate respiratory symptoms such as coughing and congestion.

Before starting any new dietary supplement regimen, it's important to consult with a healthcare professional, especially if you have pre-existing health conditions or are taking medications. Dietary supplements should complement a balanced diet and healthy lifestyle practices, including regular exercise, adequate hydration, and proper sleep hygiene, to support overall respiratory health.

Vitamin C for Respiratory Support

Vitamin C, also known as ascorbic acid, is a water-soluble vitamin that plays a crucial role in supporting respiratory health. Here's how Vitamin C can be beneficial for respiratory support:

1. **Antioxidant Protection**: Vitamin C is a powerful antioxidant that helps protect the respiratory tract from oxidative stress caused by free radicals. By neutralizing harmful molecules, Vitamin C helps reduce inflammation and damage to lung tissue, supporting overall respiratory function.

2. **Immune Support**: Vitamin C is essential for the proper functioning of the immune system. It enhances the production and function of white blood cells, which are important for fighting off infections, including those affecting the respiratory system. Adequate Vitamin C intake may help reduce the severity and duration of respiratory infections such as colds and flu.

3. **Collagen Synthesis**: Vitamin C is necessary for the synthesis of collagen, a protein that provides structural support to the respiratory tract. Collagen helps maintain the integrity of the airway walls and

prevents damage, contributing to healthy lung function and reducing the risk of respiratory issues.

4. Mucus Production: Vitamin C plays a role in the production and secretion of mucus, which helps trap and eliminate pathogens and irritants from the respiratory tract. Adequate Vitamin C levels support the proper functioning of mucous membranes, reducing the risk of respiratory infections and promoting respiratory comfort.

5. Histamine Regulation: Vitamin C may help regulate histamine levels in the body, which are involved in allergic reactions and respiratory conditions such as asthma. By modulating histamine release, Vitamin C may help alleviate allergy-related respiratory symptoms and improve breathing.

6. Antiviral Properties: Vitamin C exhibits antiviral properties that may help inhibit the replication of respiratory viruses such as the common cold virus and influenza virus. Supplementing with Vitamin C during periods of increased respiratory infection risk may help bolster the body's defenses against viral pathogens.

7. **Reduced Severity of Symptoms**: Studies have shown that Vitamin C supplementation may reduce the severity of respiratory symptoms, including coughing, congestion, and wheezing, particularly during cold and flu season or in individuals with asthma or chronic obstructive pulmonary disease (COPD).

Vitamin C can be obtained from dietary sources such as citrus fruits, strawberries, kiwi, bell peppers, broccoli, and spinach. However, supplementation may be beneficial, especially for individuals at risk of Vitamin C deficiency or those with increased respiratory health needs. It's important to consult with a healthcare professional before starting Vitamin C supplementation, especially if you have underlying health conditions or are taking medications. They can provide guidance on the appropriate dosage and form of Vitamin C for your specific needs.

Vitamin D for Respiratory Support

Vitamin D, often referred to as the "sunshine vitamin," plays a vital role in supporting respiratory health. Here's how Vitamin D can benefit respiratory function:

1. **Immune Modulation**: Vitamin D plays a crucial role in regulating the immune system, including the innate and adaptive immune responses. Adequate Vitamin D levels are associated with enhanced immune function, which helps the body defend against respiratory infections caused by viruses and bacteria.

2. **Antiviral Properties**: Vitamin D exhibits antiviral effects against respiratory pathogens, including influenza viruses and coronaviruses. It may help reduce the risk of respiratory infections and mitigate the severity of symptoms by inhibiting viral replication and modulating the immune response.

3. **Anti-inflammatory Effects**: Vitamin D has anti-inflammatory properties that help reduce inflammation in the respiratory tract. Chronic inflammation is associated with respiratory conditions such as asthma and chronic obstructive pulmonary disease (COPD). Adequate Vitamin D levels may help alleviate inflammation and improve respiratory function.

4. **Muscle Function**: Vitamin D is essential for muscle health and function, including the muscles involved in respiration. Optimal Vitamin D levels

support respiratory muscle strength and endurance, which are important for efficient breathing and lung function.

5. **Lung Development and Repair**: Vitamin D plays a role in lung development and repair processes. Adequate Vitamin D levels during pregnancy and early childhood may contribute to optimal lung growth and function, reducing the risk of respiratory issues later in life.

6. **Modulation of Airway Smooth Muscle**: Vitamin D helps regulate the contraction and relaxation of airway smooth muscle cells. In conditions such as asthma, where airway constriction and bronchospasm occur, Vitamin D may help modulate smooth muscle tone and improve airflow.

7. **Seasonal Variation**: Vitamin D levels tend to decrease during the winter months when sunlight exposure is limited. This seasonal variation may contribute to an increased risk of respiratory infections during the colder months. Supplementing with Vitamin D during winter may help maintain optimal levels and support respiratory health.

8. **Respiratory Infections**: Low Vitamin D levels have been associated with an increased risk of respiratory infections, including the common cold, flu, and pneumonia. Supplementing with Vitamin D may help reduce the incidence and severity of respiratory infections, particularly in individuals with Vitamin D deficiency.

To maintain optimal Vitamin D levels, it's important to get regular sun exposure, consume Vitamin D-rich foods such as fatty fish, fortified dairy products, and eggs, and consider supplementation if necessary, especially during winter months or for individuals with limited sun exposure. However, it's essential to consult with a healthcare professional before starting Vitamin D supplementation, as excessive intake can lead to toxicity. They can recommend the appropriate dosage and monitor Vitamin D levels to ensure safety and efficacy.

Magnesium for Respiratory Support

Magnesium is an essential mineral that plays a crucial role in various physiological processes in the body, including respiratory function. Here's how magnesium can support respiratory health:

1. **Bronchodilation**: Magnesium helps relax the smooth muscles of the airways, leading to bronchodilation. This effect can improve airflow and alleviate symptoms of respiratory conditions such as asthma, where airway constriction (bronchoconstriction) is a common feature.

2. **Anti-inflammatory Effects**: Magnesium exhibits anti-inflammatory properties that may help reduce airway inflammation in respiratory conditions like asthma and chronic obstructive pulmonary disease (COPD). By mitigating inflammation, magnesium can contribute to improved lung function and respiratory comfort.

3. **Modulation of Calcium**: Magnesium regulates calcium levels in the body, which is important for muscle contraction, including the muscles involved in respiration. Maintaining the balance between magnesium and calcium helps ensure proper muscle function and may prevent respiratory muscle dysfunction.

4. **Support for Diaphragmatic Function**: The diaphragm is the primary muscle involved in breathing. Magnesium supports diaphragmatic function by promoting muscle relaxation and

preventing cramping or spasms, which can interfere with normal breathing patterns.

5. **Oxygen Uptake and Delivery**: Magnesium is involved in the regulation of oxygen uptake and delivery to tissues. Adequate magnesium levels support efficient oxygen transport in the bloodstream, ensuring that oxygen is adequately supplied to the respiratory system and other organs.

6. **Reduction of Bronchial Reactivity**: Magnesium supplementation may help reduce bronchial reactivity, which is the tendency of the airways to constrict in response to triggers such as allergens or irritants. By stabilizing airway tone, magnesium can help prevent asthma exacerbations and improve respiratory function.

7. **Stress Reduction**: Magnesium has calming effects on the nervous system and may help reduce stress and anxiety, which can exacerbate respiratory symptoms in individuals with conditions like asthma. By promoting relaxation, magnesium may indirectly support respiratory health.

8. **Antioxidant Activity**: Magnesium exhibits antioxidant properties that help protect lung tissue

from oxidative stress and damage caused by free radicals. By scavenging harmful molecules, magnesium may help prevent inflammation and tissue injury in the respiratory tract.

Magnesium can be obtained from dietary sources such as green leafy vegetables, nuts, seeds, whole grains, and legumes. Additionally, magnesium supplements are available in various forms, including magnesium citrate, magnesium glycinate, and magnesium oxide. It's important to consult with a healthcare professional before starting magnesium supplementation, especially if you have underlying health conditions or are taking medications. They can recommend the appropriate dosage and form of magnesium based on your individual needs and monitor for any potential interactions or side effects.

Omega-3 Fatty Acids for Respiratory Support

Omega-3 fatty acids are a group of polyunsaturated fats that are essential for overall health, including respiratory function. Here's how omega-3 fatty acids can support respiratory health:

1. **Anti-inflammatory Effects**: Omega-3 fatty acids, particularly eicosapentaenoic acid (EPA) and docosahexaenoic acid (DHA), have potent anti-inflammatory properties. In respiratory conditions such as asthma and chronic obstructive pulmonary disease (COPD), inflammation of the airways contributes to symptoms such as wheezing and breathlessness. Omega-3 fatty acids help reduce airway inflammation, leading to improved lung function and respiratory comfort.

2. **Bronchodilation**: EPA and DHA have been shown to promote bronchodilation, the widening of the airways, which helps improve airflow in individuals with respiratory conditions like asthma. By relaxing the smooth muscles of the airways, omega-3 fatty acids alleviate bronchoconstriction and facilitate easier breathing.

3. **Mucus Regulation**: Omega-3 fatty acids help regulate mucus production in the respiratory tract. In conditions such as asthma and chronic bronchitis, excessive mucus production can contribute to airway obstruction and exacerbate symptoms. Omega-3 fatty acids promote a healthy balance of mucus production, reducing congestion and promoting clear airways.

4. **Immune Modulation**: Omega-3 fatty acids play a role in modulating the immune response, including the inflammatory response to respiratory infections. By regulating immune function, omega-3 fatty acids may help reduce the risk of respiratory infections and mitigate their severity and duration.

5. **Antioxidant Activity**: Omega-3 fatty acids have antioxidant properties that help protect lung tissue from oxidative stress and damage caused by free radicals. By neutralizing harmful molecules, omega-3 fatty acids help prevent inflammation and tissue injury in the respiratory tract.

6. **Improved Lung Function**: Studies have shown that omega-3 fatty acid supplementation may improve lung function parameters such as forced expiratory volume in one second (FEV1) and forced vital capacity (FVC) in individuals with respiratory conditions like asthma and COPD. Improved lung function results in better respiratory efficiency and reduced symptoms.

7. **Cardiovascular Health Benefits**: Omega-3 fatty acids have cardiovascular benefits, including reducing the risk of heart disease and stroke. Cardiovascular health is closely linked to

respiratory health, as adequate blood flow and oxygen delivery are essential for optimal lung function.

Omega-3 fatty acids are primarily found in fatty fish such as salmon, mackerel, and sardines, as well as in plant sources like flaxseeds, chia seeds, and walnuts. Additionally, omega-3 supplements, such as fish oil or algae oil capsules, are available for individuals who may not consume enough omega-3-rich foods. It's important to consult with a healthcare professional before starting omega-3 supplementation, especially if you have underlying health conditions or are taking medications. They can recommend the appropriate dosage and form of omega-3 fatty acids based on your individual needs and monitor for any potential interactions or side effects.

Quercetin for Respiratory Support

Quercetin is a flavonoid found in various fruits, vegetables, and plant-based foods. It is known for its antioxidant, anti-inflammatory, and antiviral properties, which can support respiratory health in several ways:

1. **Anti-inflammatory Effects**: Quercetin has potent anti-inflammatory properties that help reduce inflammation in the respiratory tract. In conditions such as asthma and chronic obstructive pulmonary disease (COPD), inflammation contributes to airway constriction and respiratory symptoms. Quercetin helps alleviate inflammation, leading to improved lung function and respiratory comfort.

2. **Antioxidant Activity**: Quercetin acts as an antioxidant, scavenging free radicals and protecting lung tissue from oxidative stress and damage. By neutralizing harmful molecules, quercetin helps prevent inflammation and tissue injury in the respiratory tract, promoting overall respiratory health.

3. **Bronchodilation**: Quercetin has been shown to promote bronchodilation, the widening of the airways, which helps improve airflow in individuals with respiratory conditions like asthma. By relaxing the smooth muscles of the airways, quercetin alleviates bronchoconstriction and facilitates easier breathing.

4. **Antiviral Properties**: Quercetin exhibits antiviral effects against respiratory viruses such as

the common cold virus and influenza virus. It may help reduce the risk of respiratory infections and mitigate the severity of symptoms by inhibiting viral replication and modulating the immune response.

5. **Allergy Relief**: Quercetin may help alleviate allergy-related respiratory symptoms such as sneezing, runny nose, and nasal congestion. It acts as a natural antihistamine, inhibiting the release of histamine and other inflammatory compounds that contribute to allergic reactions in the respiratory tract.

6. **Immune Modulation**: Quercetin helps modulate the immune response, including the inflammatory response to respiratory infections. By regulating immune function, quercetin may help reduce the risk of respiratory infections and enhance the body's ability to fight off pathogens.

7. **Mucolytic Activity**: Quercetin may help thin and loosen mucus in the respiratory tract, making it easier to expel. This can be beneficial for individuals with conditions such as bronchitis and chronic sinusitis, where excessive mucus production contributes to congestion and respiratory symptoms.

Quercetin-rich foods include apples, onions, citrus fruits, berries, leafy greens, and red grapes. Additionally, quercetin supplements are available in various forms, including capsules, tablets, and powders. It's important to consult with a healthcare professional before starting quercetin supplementation, especially if you have underlying health conditions or are taking medications. They can recommend the appropriate dosage and form of quercetin based on your individual needs and monitor for any potential interactions or side effects.

Chapter 7

Breathing Exercises and Techniques

Breathing exercises and techniques can be beneficial for improving respiratory function, reducing stress, and promoting overall well-being. Here are some effective breathing exercises and techniques for respiratory support:

1. **Diaphragmatic Breathing (Belly Breathing)**:
   - Sit or lie down in a comfortable position.
   - Place one hand on your abdomen and the other on your chest.
   - Inhale deeply through your nose, allowing your abdomen to rise while keeping your chest relatively still.
   - Exhale slowly through your mouth, gently contracting your abdominal muscles to expel air.
   - Focus on breathing deeply into your diaphragm, allowing your lungs to fully expand and contract with each breath.

2. **Pursed Lip Breathing**:
   - Inhale deeply through your nose.
   - Purse your lips as if you're about to whistle.

- Exhale slowly and gently through pursed lips, as if you're blowing out a candle.
- The resistance created by pursing your lips helps slow down your breathing and keeps airways open longer, improving oxygen exchange.

3. **Box Breathing (Square Breathing)**:
   - Inhale deeply through your nose to a count of four.
   - Hold your breath for a count of four.
   - Exhale slowly and completely through your mouth to a count of four.
   - Hold your breath for a count of four before inhaling again.
   - Repeat the cycle for several rounds, focusing on the rhythmic pattern of inhaling, holding, exhaling, and holding.

4. **Alternate Nostril Breathing (Nadi Shodhana)**:
   - Sit comfortably with your spine straight.
   - Close your right nostril with your right thumb and inhale deeply through your left nostril.
   - Close your left nostril with your ring finger and exhale completely through your right nostril.
   - Inhale through your right nostril, then close it with your thumb and exhale through your left nostril.

- Continue alternating nostrils for several rounds, maintaining a steady breath and focusing on the sensation of air flowing in and out of each nostril.

5. **4-7-8 Breathing**:
   - Inhale deeply through your nose to a count of four.
   - Hold your breath for a count of seven.
   - Exhale slowly and completely through your mouth to a count of eight, making a whooshing sound.
   - Repeat the cycle for several rounds, allowing each exhalation to be longer than the inhalation.

6. **Resonant Breathing**:
   - Find a comfortable breathing rhythm and focus on the natural resonance of your breath.
   - Inhale and exhale smoothly and evenly, without forcing or straining.
   - Imagine your breath resonating in a specific area of your body, such as your chest or abdomen.
   - Maintain a steady and relaxed breathing pattern, allowing the resonance to deepen with each breath.

Practice these breathing exercises regularly to improve lung function, reduce stress, and enhance overall respiratory health. Incorporating deep breathing into your daily routine can help increase oxygenation, relax tense muscles, and promote a sense of calm and well-being. If you have any respiratory conditions or concerns, consult with a healthcare professional before starting a new breathing exercise regimen.

Diaphragmatic Breathing (Belly Breathing):

Diaphragmatic breathing, also known as belly breathing, is a technique that involves engaging the diaphragm, the primary muscle responsible for breathing, to promote efficient and deep breathing. Here's how to practice diaphragmatic breathing:

1. **Find a Comfortable Position**: Sit or lie down in a comfortable position, with your back straight and your shoulders relaxed. You can place one hand on your abdomen and the other on your chest to feel the movement of your breath.

2. **Relax Your Shoulders**: Allow your shoulders to relax and avoid tensing them as you breathe. Keep your chest relatively still while focusing on breathing deeply into your abdomen.

3. **Inhale Slowly and Deeply**: Inhale through your nose slowly and deeply, allowing your

abdomen to rise as you fill your lungs with air. Feel your diaphragm expanding downward into your abdomen.

4. **Exhale Completely**: Exhale slowly and completely through your mouth or nose, gently contracting your abdominal muscles to expel air. Feel your abdomen fall as you empty your lungs.

5. **Focus on Your Breath**: Pay attention to the sensation of your breath as it moves in and out of your body. Focus on the rhythm of your breath and the movement of your abdomen with each inhalation and exhalation.

6. **Repeat**: Continue to inhale deeply into your abdomen and exhale completely, maintaining a slow and steady rhythm of breathing. Aim to practice diaphragmatic breathing for several minutes, gradually increasing the duration as you become more comfortable with the technique.

Benefits of Diaphragmatic Breathing:
- **Improves Lung Function**: Diaphragmatic breathing helps maximize the use of your lung capacity, allowing for more efficient oxygen exchange and carbon dioxide elimination.

- **Reduces Stress and Anxiety**: Deep breathing activates the body's relaxation response, promoting feelings of calm and reducing stress and anxiety.
- **Promotes Relaxation**: Diaphragmatic breathing can help relax tense muscles, lower blood pressure, and alleviate physical symptoms of stress.
- **Enhances Focus and Concentration**: Deep breathing exercises can improve mental clarity and focus by increasing oxygen flow to the brain.

Incorporate diaphragmatic breathing into your daily routine, especially during times of stress or when you need to relax and unwind. With regular practice, diaphragmatic breathing can become a natural and effortless way to support your respiratory health and overall well-being.

Pursed Lip Breathing:

Pursed lip breathing is a breathing technique that can help improve breathing efficiency, reduce shortness of breath, and promote relaxation. It involves inhaling through the nose and exhaling slowly through pursed lips, creating resistance to the airflow. Here's how to practice pursed lip breathing:

1. **Find a Comfortable Position**: Sit or stand in a comfortable position with your back straight and shoulders relaxed. You can place one hand on your abdomen to feel the movement of your breath.

2. **Inhale Slowly Through Your Nose**: Take a slow, deep breath in through your nose, filling your lungs with air. Focus on breathing deeply into your abdomen, allowing it to expand as you inhale.

3. **Purse Your Lips**: Pucker or purse your lips together, as if you're about to blow out a candle or whistle.

4. **Exhale Slowly Through Pursed Lips**: Exhale slowly and gently through your pursed lips, making a slight hissing sound as you exhale. Imagine you're blowing out through a straw, maintaining gentle pressure to create resistance to the airflow.

5. **Lengthen Your Exhalation**: Focus on prolonging your exhalation, taking twice as long to exhale as you did to inhale. This slow, controlled exhalation helps reduce the feeling of breathlessness and allows for more complete air exchange in the lungs.

6. **Repeat Several Times**: Continue to inhale through your nose and exhale through pursed lips, repeating the cycle for several breaths. Aim to practice pursed lip breathing for a few minutes at a time, gradually increasing the duration as you become more comfortable with the technique.

Benefits of Pursed Lip Breathing:
- **Improves Breathing Efficiency**: Pursed lip breathing helps regulate the pace of breathing and reduces the work of breathing, making it easier to take in oxygen and expel carbon dioxide.
- **Reduces Shortness of Breath**: Pursed lip breathing can alleviate feelings of breathlessness, particularly during physical activity or periods of anxiety or stress.
- **Promotes Relaxation**: The slow, controlled exhalation of pursed lip breathing activates the body's relaxation response, promoting feelings of calm and relaxation.
- **Supports Lung Health**: Pursed lip breathing helps prevent airway collapse and maintains positive pressure in the airways, which can be beneficial for individuals with conditions such as asthma, COPD, or emphysema.

Incorporate pursed lip breathing into your daily routine, especially during times when you feel short of breath or anxious. With regular practice, pursed lip breathing can become a helpful tool for managing respiratory symptoms and promoting overall well-being.

Buteyko Breathing Technique:

The Buteyko Breathing Technique is a method developed by Russian physician Dr. Konstantin Buteyko to address breathing pattern disorders and improve respiratory health. It focuses on reducing overbreathing (hyperventilation) and promoting nasal breathing to optimize oxygenation and carbon dioxide levels in the body. Here's how to practice the Buteyko Breathing Technique:

1. **Nasal Breathing**: Buteyko emphasizes the importance of breathing through the nose rather than the mouth. Nasal breathing helps filter, humidify, and warm the air before it reaches the lungs, as well as promoting the production of nitric oxide, which supports respiratory function.

2. **Reduced Breathing**: The Buteyko technique involves consciously reducing the volume and frequency of breathing to achieve a state of slight air hunger. This is accomplished by gently slowing

down the pace of breathing and reducing the size of each breath.

3. **Controlled Exhalation**: Focus on prolonging the exhalation phase of each breath, allowing the lungs to empty fully before inhaling again. This helps prevent overinflation of the lungs and maintains a balanced exchange of oxygen and carbon dioxide.

4. **Breath Holding**: After each exhalation, hold your breath for a brief period (typically 2-5 seconds) before inhaling again. This allows carbon dioxide levels to rise slightly in the bloodstream, which helps regulate breathing and optimize oxygen delivery to tissues.

5. **Relaxation**: Practice the Buteyko Breathing Technique in a relaxed and mindful manner, focusing on the sensations of breathing and allowing tension to release from the body. Avoid forceful or exaggerated breathing, and aim for a smooth and natural rhythm of breathing.

6. **Practice Regularly**: Incorporate the Buteyko Breathing Technique into your daily routine, dedicating time each day to practice the exercises. Start with short sessions and gradually increase the

duration as you become more comfortable with the technique.

Benefits of the Buteyko Breathing Technique:

- **Improved Respiratory Function**: The Buteyko technique helps restore normal breathing patterns and optimize respiratory parameters, such as oxygen and carbon dioxide levels, lung capacity, and airway patency.
- **Reduced Symptoms**: Practicing Buteyko breathing may alleviate symptoms of respiratory conditions such as asthma, allergies, sinusitis, and sleep apnea, including shortness of breath, wheezing, congestion, and snoring.
- **Enhanced Athletic Performance**: Nasal breathing and controlled breathing techniques taught in Buteyko can benefit athletes by improving oxygenation, endurance, and recovery, as well as reducing the risk of exercise-induced asthma.
- **Stress Reduction**: Buteyko Breathing promotes relaxation, reduces sympathetic nervous system activity, and enhances parasympathetic nervous system activation, leading to decreased stress levels and improved overall well-being.

It's essential to learn the Buteyko Breathing Technique from a qualified instructor who can provide personalized guidance and support. With consistent practice and guidance, the Buteyko Breathing Technique can be a valuable tool for optimizing respiratory health and enhancing overall quality of life.

Yoga and Pranayama for Respiratory Health:

Yoga, an ancient practice originating in India, incorporates physical postures, breath control (pranayama), and meditation to promote holistic well-being. Pranayama, or yogic breathing techniques, plays a significant role in enhancing respiratory health by improving lung function, increasing oxygenation, and reducing stress. Here's how yoga and pranayama can benefit respiratory health:

1. **Deep Breathing**: Many yoga practices emphasize deep breathing techniques, such as diaphragmatic breathing and belly breathing, which help expand lung capacity, increase oxygen intake, and promote relaxation.

2. **Pranayama Techniques**:

- **Ujjayi Pranayama (Victorious Breath)**: Ujjayi breathing involves constricting the back of the throat slightly while breathing deeply through the nose, creating a subtle oceanic sound. It helps regulate breathing, increase oxygenation, and calm the mind.

- **Kapalabhati Pranayama (Skull Shining Breath)**: Kapalabhati involves forceful exhalations through the nose, followed by passive inhalations. This energizing breath technique helps clear the nasal passages, increase lung capacity, and invigorate the body.

- **Anulom Vilom Pranayama (Alternate Nostril Breathing)**: Anulom Vilom involves alternating nostril breathing, where you inhale through one nostril while closing the other nostril with your thumb, then exhale through the opposite nostril while closing the other nostril with your ring finger. This balances the flow of energy in the body, promotes mental clarity, and supports respiratory function.

3. **Yoga Asanas (Poses)**: Certain yoga postures can help open up the chest, improve posture, and enhance lung function. Poses such as Cobra Pose (Bhujangasana), Bridge Pose (Setu Bandhasana), and Fish Pose (Matsyasana) stretch the chest

muscles, expand the rib cage, and increase lung capacity.

4. **Mindfulness and Relaxation**: Yoga practice often incorporates mindfulness techniques and relaxation exercises, such as Savasana (Corpse Pose) and Yoga Nidra (Yogic Sleep), which help reduce stress, calm the nervous system, and promote deep relaxation, allowing for better respiratory function.

5. **Stress Reduction**: Chronic stress can negatively impact respiratory health by exacerbating conditions such as asthma and COPD. Yoga and pranayama help reduce stress levels, lower cortisol levels, and promote a sense of well-being, which can positively affect respiratory function.

6. **Improved Breathing Patterns**: Regular practice of yoga and pranayama helps cultivate awareness of breathing patterns and encourages more efficient, diaphragmatic breathing, leading to better oxygenation and ventilation of the lungs.

Incorporating yoga and pranayama into your daily routine can provide numerous benefits for respiratory health, including improved lung function, reduced stress, and enhanced overall well-being. It's essential to practice under the guidance of a qualified yoga instructor, especially if you have underlying health conditions or specific respiratory concerns. With consistent practice and mindfulness, yoga and pranayama can become valuable tools for supporting respiratory health and promoting a balanced and harmonious life.

Chapter 8

Steam Therapy and Humidification for Respiratory Health:

Steam therapy and humidification are techniques used to moisten and warm the airways, loosen mucus, and provide relief from respiratory symptoms such as congestion, coughing, and dryness. Here's how steam therapy and humidification can benefit respiratory health:

1. **Moisturizes the Airways**: Dry air can irritate the respiratory tract and exacerbate symptoms of respiratory conditions such as asthma, allergies, and sinusitis. Steam therapy and humidification add moisture to the air, keeping the airways hydrated and reducing irritation.

2. **Loosens Mucus**: Steam inhalation helps loosen and thin mucus in the respiratory tract, making it easier to expel. This can provide relief from congestion, coughing, and nasal congestion associated with respiratory infections or conditions such as bronchitis and COPD.

3. **Facilitates Breathing**: Breathing in warm, moist air can help open up the airways and improve

breathing efficiency, especially in individuals with conditions characterized by airway constriction, such as asthma and chronic bronchitis.

4. **Relieves Nasal Congestion**: Steam therapy can help relieve nasal congestion and sinus pressure by moisturizing the nasal passages and promoting drainage of mucus. This can alleviate symptoms of sinusitis, allergies, and colds.

5. **Soothes Irritated Airways**: Steam inhalation has a soothing effect on the respiratory tract, providing relief from throat irritation, dry cough, and soreness. It can also help alleviate symptoms of laryngitis and other respiratory conditions affecting the throat.

6. **Promotes Relaxation**: Steam therapy and humidification can have a calming effect on the body and mind, promoting relaxation and reducing stress levels. This can be beneficial for individuals experiencing respiratory symptoms exacerbated by stress or anxiety.

Ways to Incorporate Steam Therapy and Humidification:

1. **Steam Inhalation**: Fill a bowl with hot water and add a few drops of essential oils (such as eucalyptus or peppermint) if desired. Lean over the bowl, covering your head with a towel to trap the steam, and inhale deeply for 5-10 minutes. Be cautious to avoid burns from the hot steam.

2. **Humidifiers**: Use a humidifier to add moisture to the air in your home, especially during dry winter months or in arid climates. Cool mist or warm mist humidifiers are available, depending on personal preference and needs.

3. **Steam Shower or Bath**: Take a steamy shower or bath to benefit from the steam and humidity. Breathing in the warm, moist air can help alleviate congestion and promote relaxation.

4. **Nebulizers**: Nebulizers are devices that convert liquid medication into a fine mist, which can be inhaled directly into the lungs. They are often used to administer medications for respiratory conditions such as asthma and COPD.

5. **Hydration**: In addition to steam therapy and humidification, staying well-hydrated by drinking plenty of fluids can help keep the respiratory tract moist and facilitate mucus clearance.

While steam therapy and humidification can provide relief from respiratory symptoms, it's essential to use them safely and appropriately to avoid potential risks, such as burns or mold growth. Follow manufacturer instructions for humidifier use, and consult with a healthcare professional if you have any underlying health conditions or concerns about steam therapy.

Steam Inhalation for Respiratory Health:

Steam inhalation is a simple and effective home remedy for alleviating respiratory symptoms, clearing nasal passages, and soothing irritated airways. It involves inhaling warm, moist air to moisturize the respiratory tract, loosen mucus, and provide relief from congestion, coughing, and sinus discomfort. Here's how to practice steam inhalation safely and effectively:

1. **Boil Water**: Bring a pot or kettle of water to a boil on the stove. You can also use a heatproof bowl or basin filled with hot water.

2. **Optional: Add Essential Oils**: For added benefits, you can add a few drops of essential oils to the hot water. Eucalyptus, peppermint, and tea tree oil are commonly used for their decongestant, antiviral, and antibacterial properties. However, be cautious not to use too much oil, as it can irritate sensitive airways.

3. **Create a Tent**: Carefully transfer the hot water to a heatproof surface, such as a table or countertop. Sit comfortably with your head positioned over the steaming water, but at a safe distance to avoid burns. You can create a tent by draping a towel over your head and the pot or basin to trap the steam.

4. **Inhale Deeply**: Close your eyes and inhale deeply through your nose, allowing the warm steam to enter your nasal passages and lungs. Breathe slowly and steadily, focusing on the sensation of the steam opening up your airways.

5. **Exhale Slowly**: After inhaling deeply, exhale slowly through your mouth, releasing any tension

or congestion in your chest. Continue to inhale and exhale deeply for 5-10 minutes, or until you feel relief from respiratory symptoms.

6. **Be Cautious**: Take care not to get too close to the hot water to avoid burns. If the steam feels too hot or uncomfortable, move farther away or take a break until it cools slightly. Children should be supervised during steam inhalation to prevent accidents.

7. **Stay Hydrated**: Drink plenty of water before and after steam inhalation to stay hydrated and help thin mucus in the respiratory tract.

Steam inhalation can be repeated several times a day as needed to relieve congestion and respiratory discomfort. It's a safe and natural remedy that can complement other treatments for respiratory conditions such as colds, sinus infections, allergies, and bronchitis. However, if you have severe respiratory symptoms or underlying health conditions, it's essential to consult with a healthcare professional before using steam inhalation.

Humidifiers and Vaporizers for Respiratory Health:

Humidifiers and vaporizers are devices designed to increase moisture levels in the air, which can provide relief from respiratory symptoms and improve overall respiratory health. While both devices add humidity to the air, they operate differently and serve distinct purposes. Here's an overview of humidifiers and vaporizers and their benefits for respiratory health:

Humidifiers:

1. **Purpose**: Humidifiers are designed to add moisture to the air to increase humidity levels in indoor environments, particularly during dry weather conditions or in regions with low humidity.

2. **Types**:
   - **Cool Mist Humidifiers**: These humidifiers use a fan to evaporate water into the air, creating a cool mist. They are ideal for adding moisture to the air without raising the room temperature.
   - **Warm Mist Humidifiers**: Warm mist humidifiers boil water to produce steam, which is then released into the air. They can help kill

bacteria and viruses in the water, making them suitable for individuals with respiratory infections.

  - **Ultrasonic Humidifiers**: Ultrasonic humidifiers use ultrasonic vibrations to produce a fine mist of water droplets, which is then released into the air. They are quiet and energy-efficient, making them suitable for use in bedrooms and nurseries.

3. **Benefits**:
  - **Relieves Dryness**: Humidifiers can alleviate symptoms of dry air, such as dry throat, nasal congestion, coughing, and irritated airways.
  - **Moisturizes Respiratory Tract**: Increased humidity helps moisturize the respiratory tract, keeping mucous membranes hydrated and reducing irritation.
  - **Supports Healing**: Humidifiers can promote faster healing of respiratory conditions such as colds, sinusitis, and bronchitis by creating a moist environment that supports the body's natural healing processes.

Vaporizers:

1. **Purpose**: Vaporizers are devices that heat water to produce steam or vapor, which is then released

into the air to increase humidity levels and provide therapeutic benefits.

2. **Types**:
   - **Steam Vaporizers**: These devices boil water to produce steam, which is then released into the air. They are effective for adding moisture to the air and can help alleviate respiratory symptoms such as congestion and coughing.
   - **Ultrasonic Vaporizers**: Similar to ultrasonic humidifiers, ultrasonic vaporizers use ultrasonic vibrations to produce a fine mist of water vapor. They are quiet and efficient, making them suitable for use in bedrooms and other quiet environments.

3. **Benefits**:
   - Relieves Congestion: Vaporizers can help relieve nasal congestion and sinus pressure by moisturizing the nasal passages and promoting mucus drainage.
   - **Soothes Irritation**: The warm, moist air produced by vaporizers can soothe irritated airways and throat, providing relief from coughing, sore throat, and dryness.
   - **Facilitates Relaxation**: Vaporizers create a comforting and relaxing environment, which can promote better sleep and overall respiratory comfort.

Safety Tips:
- Follow manufacturer instructions for proper use and maintenance of humidifiers and vaporizers to prevent mold growth and bacterial contamination.
- Use distilled or filtered water to avoid mineral buildup and reduce the risk of spreading impurities into the air.
- Clean and disinfect humidifier and vaporizer components regularly to prevent bacterial growth and maintain air quality.
- Keep humidifiers and vaporizers out of reach of children and pets, and use caution when handling hot water or steam.

In summary, humidifiers and vaporizers are valuable tools for maintaining optimal humidity levels in indoor environments and promoting respiratory health. By adding moisture to the air, these devices can provide relief from dry air symptoms, alleviate respiratory congestion, and support overall respiratory comfort. However, it's essential to choose the right type of device and use it safely and appropriately to maximize its benefits and minimize potential risks. If you have any respiratory conditions or concerns, consult with a healthcare professional before using a humidifier or vaporizer.

Herbal Steam Blends for Respiratory Health:

Herbal steam blends are natural remedies that utilize the therapeutic properties of aromatic herbs to provide relief from respiratory symptoms, such as congestion, coughing, and sinus discomfort. Steam inhalation with herbal blends can help moisturize the airways, loosen mucus, and soothe irritated respiratory tissues. Here are some common herbs used in steam blends for respiratory health:

1. **Eucalyptus**:
   - **Benefits**: Eucalyptus has decongestant, expectorant, and antimicrobial properties, making it effective for clearing nasal passages, relieving congestion, and supporting respiratory health.
   - **Usage**: Add a few drops of eucalyptus essential oil or fresh eucalyptus leaves to hot water for steam inhalation. Inhale deeply to experience the refreshing aroma and respiratory benefits of eucalyptus.

2. **Peppermint**:
   - **Benefits**: Peppermint has cooling and soothing properties that can help alleviate nasal congestion, sinus pressure, and throat irritation. It also has

antimicrobial effects, which may help combat respiratory infections.

   - **Usage**: Add dried peppermint leaves or a few drops of peppermint essential oil to hot water for steam inhalation. Inhale the invigorating aroma of peppermint to relieve congestion and promote respiratory comfort.

3. **Lavender**:
   - **Benefits**: Lavender is known for its calming and relaxing properties, which can help reduce stress, anxiety, and tension. Inhalation of lavender steam may promote relaxation and improve overall respiratory well-being.
   - **Usage**: Add dried lavender flowers or a few drops of lavender essential oil to hot water for steam inhalation. Breathe deeply to enjoy the soothing aroma of lavender and promote respiratory relaxation.

4. **Chamomile**:
   - **Benefits**: Chamomile has anti-inflammatory and antimicrobial properties that can help soothe irritated airways, reduce inflammation, and promote respiratory comfort. It may also have mild sedative effects, aiding in relaxation.
   - **Usage**: Add dried chamomile flowers or a few drops of chamomile essential oil to hot water for

steam inhalation. Inhale the gentle aroma of chamomile to soothe respiratory tissues and promote a sense of calm.

5. **Rosemary**:
   - **Benefits**: Rosemary has expectorant and antimicrobial properties that can help clear congestion, support respiratory function, and alleviate respiratory infections. It also has a stimulating aroma that can help invigorate the senses.
   - **Usage**: Add dried rosemary leaves or a few drops of rosemary essential oil to hot water for steam inhalation. Inhale deeply to experience the uplifting aroma of rosemary and promote respiratory clarity.

6. **Thyme**:
   - **Benefits**: Thyme contains compounds such as thymol, which have antiseptic, expectorant, and antimicrobial properties. Thyme steam inhalation may help clear mucus, relieve congestion, and support respiratory health.
   - **Usage**: Add dried thyme leaves or a few drops of thyme essential oil to hot water for steam inhalation. Inhale the aromatic steam to promote respiratory comfort and clarity.

Usage Tips:
- Choose organic, high-quality herbs and essential oils for steam blends to ensure purity and potency.
- Use caution when adding essential oils to hot water, as they can be potent. Start with a small amount and adjust to your preference.
- Perform a patch test before using essential oils topically or inhaling them to ensure you do not have any sensitivities or allergic reactions.
- Keep your eyes closed during steam inhalation to avoid irritation from the herbal vapors.
- If you have respiratory conditions or concerns, consult with a healthcare professional before using herbal steam blends to ensure they are appropriate for your individual needs.

By incorporating herbal steam blends into your self-care routine, you can harness the natural healing properties of aromatic herbs to support respiratory health, alleviate symptoms, and promote overall well-being.

Chapter 9

Acupuncture and Acupressure Points for Respiratory Health:

Acupuncture and acupressure are traditional Chinese medicine techniques that involve stimulating specific points on the body to promote healing and relieve various ailments, including respiratory conditions. By targeting key acupoints associated with the respiratory system, these techniques can help alleviate symptoms such as coughing, wheezing, congestion, and shortness of breath. Here are some common acupuncture and acupressure points used for respiratory health:

1. **Lung Meridian (LU 1 - LU 11):**
   - **LU 1 (Zhongfu - Central Residence):** Located on the upper chest, approximately 1.5 inches below the collarbone, in the depression below the clavicle. Stimulating this point can help open the chest, relieve congestion, and promote deep breathing.
   - **LU 5 (Chize - Cubit Marsh):** Located on the forearm, approximately 1.5 inches above the wrist crease, on the radial side of the tendon of the biceps brachii muscle. Stimulating this point can help relieve coughing, wheezing, and asthma symptoms.

- **LU 9 (Taiyuan - Great Abyss)**: Located on the wrist crease, in the depression between the radial artery and the tendon of the abductor pollicis longus muscle. Stimulating this point can help tonify lung qi, regulate breathing, and alleviate respiratory discomfort.

2. **Large Intestine Meridian (LI 4 - LI 20)**:
   - **LI 4 (Hegu - Joining Valley)**: Located on the back of the hand, in the webbing between the thumb and index finger. Stimulating this point can help disperse lung qi, relieve nasal congestion, and alleviate sinusitis symptoms.
   - **LI 20 (Yingxiang - Welcome Fragrance)**: Located on the sides of the nostrils, at the level of the midpoint of the nasolabial groove. Stimulating this point can help open nasal passages, clear congestion, and promote easier breathing.

3. **Ren Meridian (CV 17)**:
   - **CV 17 (Shanzhong - Chest Center)**: Located on the midline of the chest, at the level of the fourth intercostal space, approximately 4 inches above the umbilicus. Stimulating this point can help regulate lung qi, relieve chest tightness, and promote deep breathing.

4. **Governing Vessel Meridian (GV 14)**:
   - **GV 14 (Dazhui - Great Vertebrae)**: Located on the midline of the back, in the depression below the spinous process of the seventh cervical vertebra. Stimulating this point can help tonify lung qi, relieve coughing, and alleviate respiratory congestion.

5. **Stomach Meridian (ST 36)**:
   - **ST 36 (Zusanli - Leg Three Miles)**: Located on the lower leg, approximately 3 inches below the knee, on the lateral side of the shinbone. Stimulating this point can help tonify lung qi, boost immune function, and improve overall respiratory health.

Acupuncture involves the insertion of thin needles into specific acupoints, while acupressure involves applying pressure to these points using fingers, thumbs, or specialized tools. Both techniques can be effective for promoting respiratory health and relieving respiratory symptoms when performed by a qualified practitioner.

It's essential to consult with a licensed acupuncturist or qualified healthcare professional before undergoing acupuncture or acupressure treatment, especially if you have underlying health conditions or concerns. They can provide personalized recommendations and ensure that the treatment is safe and appropriate for your individual needs.

The Lung Meridian in traditional Chinese medicine (TCM) consists of several acupuncture points that are believed to influence the function of the lungs and respiratory system. These points are strategically located along the pathway of the lung meridian, which runs from the chest down to the hand. Stimulating these points through acupuncture or acupressure may help alleviate respiratory symptoms and promote lung health. Here are some key Lung Meridian points:

1. **LU 1 (Zhongfu - Central Residence)**:
   - Location: On the upper chest, approximately 1.5 inches below the collarbone, in the depression below the clavicle.
   - Benefits: Stimulating this point can help open the chest, relieve congestion, and promote deep breathing.

2. **LU 5 (Chize - Cubit Marsh)**:
   - Location: On the forearm, approximately 1.5 inches above the wrist crease, on the radial side of the tendon of the biceps brachii muscle.

- Benefits: Stimulating this point can help relieve coughing, wheezing, and asthma symptoms.

3. **LU 9 (Taiyuan - Great Abyss)**:
  - Location: On the wrist crease, in the depression between the radial artery and the tendon of the abductor pollicis longus muscle.
  - Benefits: Stimulating this point can help tonify lung qi, regulate breathing, and alleviate respiratory discomfort.

4. **LU 10 (Yuji - Fish Border)**:
  - Location: On the palm side of the hand, in the webbing between the thumb and index finger, at the midpoint of the first metacarpal bone.
  - Benefits: Stimulating this point can help clear lung heat, reduce fever, and alleviate sore throat.

5. **LU 11 (Shaoshang - Lesser Shang)**:
  - Location: At the tip of the thumb, on the radial side of the nail.
  - Benefits: Stimulating this point can help clear lung heat, reduce inflammation, and alleviate sore throat and coughing.

These are just a few of the key acupuncture points along the Lung Meridian. In traditional Chinese medicine, the lung meridian is considered to be closely connected to the respiratory system, as well as the skin, immune system, and emotions. By stimulating these points, practitioners aim to restore balance and harmony within the body, thereby promoting overall health and well-being.

The Conception Vessel Meridian, also known as the Ren Meridian in traditional Chinese medicine (TCM), is a significant energy pathway in the body that runs along the midline of the front of the body. It is associated with the regulation of qi (vital energy) and the circulation of blood, as well as the nourishment of the organs and tissues. Stimulating specific points along the Conception Vessel Meridian can help address various health issues and promote overall well-being. Here are some key Conception Vessel Meridian points:

1. **CV 1 (Huiyin - Meeting of Yin)**:
   - Location: At the perineum, between the anus and the genitals.
   - Benefits: Stimulating this point can help tonify the kidneys, regulate menstruation, and strengthen the lower back.

2. **CV 4 (Guanyuan - Gate of Origin)**:
   - Location: On the midline of the lower abdomen, approximately three finger widths below the navel.
   - Benefits: Stimulating this point can help tonify the spleen and stomach, regulate digestion, and nourish the body's qi and blood.

3. **CV 6 (Qihai - Sea of Qi)**:
   - Location: On the midline of the lower abdomen, approximately one and a half inches below the navel.
   - Benefits: Stimulating this point can help tonify the body's qi and blood, strengthen the immune system, and regulate menstruation.

4. **CV 12 (Zhongwan - Middle Cavity)**:
   - Location: On the midline of the upper abdomen, approximately four finger widths above the navel.
   - Benefits: Stimulating this point can help regulate digestion, alleviate nausea and vomiting, and tonify the spleen and stomach.

5. **CV 17 (Shanzhong - Chest Center)**:
   - Location: On the midline of the chest, at the level of the fourth intercostal space, approximately four inches above the umbilicus.

- Benefits: Stimulating this point can help regulate qi circulation in the chest, alleviate chest congestion and discomfort, and promote emotional well-being.

6. **CV 24 (Chengjiang - Connecting Channel)**:
   - Location: On the midline of the lower lip, at the junction of the upper and lower lips.
   - Benefits: Stimulating this point can help regulate the flow of qi and blood in the face and mouth, alleviate toothaches, and promote oral health.

These are just a few of the key Conception Vessel Meridian points. Stimulating these points through acupuncture, acupressure, or other traditional Chinese medicine techniques can help balance the body's energy, promote health, and alleviate various health issues. It's essential to consult with a qualified practitioner of traditional Chinese medicine for personalized recommendations and treatment.

The Governing Vessel Meridian, also known as the Du Meridian in traditional Chinese medicine (TCM), is a major energy pathway that runs along the midline of the back and the head. It is closely associated with the central nervous system, the spine, and the brain. Stimulating specific points along the Governing Vessel Meridian can help regulate the flow of qi (vital energy) and blood, balance yin and yang energies, and promote overall health and well-being. Here are some key Governing Vessel Meridian points:

1. GV 14 (Dazhui - Great Vertebrae):
   - Location: On the midline of the upper back, in the depression below the spinous process of the seventh cervical vertebra (C7).
   - Benefits: Stimulating this point can help regulate qi circulation in the upper back, alleviate neck and shoulder tension, and promote relaxation.

2. GV 20 (Baihui - Hundred Meetings):
   - Location: On the midline of the scalp, approximately midway between the apex of the head and the hairline.
   - Benefits: Stimulating this point can help regulate qi circulation in the head, improve mental clarity and concentration, and promote spiritual awareness.

3. GV 24.5 (Yintang - Hall of Impression):
   - Location: On the midline of the forehead, between the eyebrows, at the level of the eyebrows' midpoint.

- Benefits: Stimulating this point can help calm the mind, alleviate stress and anxiety, and promote mental relaxation.

4. GV 26 (Renzhong - Man's Middle):
- Location: On the midline of the philtrum (the vertical groove between the nose and the upper lip).
- Benefits: Stimulating this point can help regulate qi circulation in the face, alleviate nasal congestion, and promote facial muscle relaxation.

5. GV 4 (Mingmen - Gate of Life):
- Location: On the midline of the lower back, approximately two finger widths above the waistline, at the level of the second lumbar vertebra (L2).
- Benefits: Stimulating this point can help tonify kidney qi, strengthen the lower back, and support overall vitality and energy.

6. GV 12 (Shenzhu - Spirit Pillar):
- Location: On the midline of the upper back, in the depression below the spinous process of the third thoracic vertebra (T3).
- Benefits: Stimulating this point can help regulate qi circulation in the upper back, alleviate shoulder tension, and promote emotional balance.

These are just a few of the key Governing Vessel Meridian points. Stimulating these points through acupuncture, acupressure, or other traditional Chinese medicine techniques can help balance the body's energy, promote health, and alleviate various health issues. It's essential to consult with a qualified practitioner of traditional Chinese medicine for personalized recommendations and treatment.

Chapter 10

Precautions and Considerations

When considering acupuncture or acupressure for respiratory health or any other condition, it's essential to keep several precautions and considerations in mind:

1. **Consultation with Healthcare Provider**: Before undergoing acupuncture or acupressure treatment, especially if you have underlying health conditions or concerns, it's crucial to consult with your primary healthcare provider. They can provide valuable insights into whether these treatments are suitable for you and whether they may interact with any medications or therapies you're currently receiving.

2. **Qualified Practitioners**: Choose a qualified and licensed acupuncturist or acupressure therapist who has received proper training and certification in traditional Chinese medicine techniques. This ensures that you receive safe and effective treatment tailored to your individual needs.

3. **Allergies and Sensitivities**: Inform your practitioner of any allergies or sensitivities you may have to certain herbs, essential oils, or acupuncture materials. This helps them customize your treatment plan and avoid potential adverse reactions.

4. **Pregnancy**: If you are pregnant or trying to conceive, discuss acupuncture or acupressure with your obstetrician or midwife before proceeding. While these techniques are generally considered safe during pregnancy, certain acupuncture points should be avoided to prevent miscarriage or premature labor.

5. **Medical Devices**: If you have medical devices implanted in your body, such as pacemakers or insulin pumps, inform your acupuncturist or acupressure therapist. Some acupuncture points may interfere with the functioning of these devices, so your practitioner can modify the treatment accordingly.

6. **Infections and Open Wounds**: Avoid acupuncture or acupressure treatment on areas with infections, open wounds, or skin lesions. Infections can spread through needle punctures,

and applying pressure to open wounds can increase the risk of infection.

7. **Discomfort or Pain**: Acupuncture and acupressure should not cause significant pain or discomfort. If you experience excessive pain, discomfort, or unusual sensations during treatment, inform your practitioner immediately.

8. **Hygiene and Safety**: Ensure that your acupuncturist or acupressure therapist follows strict hygiene practices and uses sterile needles and equipment for each session. This reduces the risk of infection and ensures your safety during treatment.

9. **Consistency and Follow-up**: For optimal results, follow your practitioner's recommendations for the frequency and duration of acupuncture or acupressure sessions. Be consistent with your treatment plan and attend follow-up appointments as advised to monitor your progress and adjust the treatment as needed.

By considering these precautions and consulting with qualified healthcare professionals, you can safely and effectively incorporate acupuncture or acupressure into your respiratory health regimen to promote overall well-being and alleviate symptoms.

Consulting with your healthcare provider is a crucial step before considering any new treatment or therapy, including acupuncture or acupressure for respiratory health. Here's why it's important:

1. **Medical History**: Your healthcare provider can review your medical history, current medications, and existing health conditions to determine if acupuncture or acupressure is safe and appropriate for you. They can identify any potential contraindications or interactions with your current treatment plan.

2. **Underlying Conditions**: If you have respiratory conditions such as asthma, COPD, or allergies, your healthcare provider can assess your specific needs and recommend complementary therapies that align with your overall treatment goals. They can provide guidance on how acupuncture or acupressure may fit into your existing respiratory management plan.

3. **Safety Concerns**: Your healthcare provider can address any safety concerns you may have about acupuncture or acupressure, particularly if you're pregnant, have a compromised immune system, or are at risk of bleeding disorders. They can provide

personalized advice based on your individual health status.

4. **Monitoring Progress**: Your healthcare provider can monitor your progress and track any changes in your respiratory symptoms over time. They can collaborate with your acupuncturist or acupressure therapist to ensure that your treatment plan is effective and aligned with your healthcare goals.

5. **Integrated Care**: Integrated care involves coordinating various healthcare services to provide comprehensive treatment for patients. By consulting with your healthcare provider, you can integrate acupuncture or acupressure into your overall healthcare plan, ensuring that it complements other therapies and treatments you may be receiving.

6. **Referrals**: If your healthcare provider determines that acupuncture or acupressure is not suitable for your condition or health status, they can provide alternative recommendations or referrals to other healthcare professionals who may better meet your needs.

7. **Personalized Recommendations**: Your healthcare provider can provide personalized recommendations based on your individual health history, preferences, and treatment goals. They can help you make informed decisions about incorporating acupuncture or acupressure into your respiratory health regimen.

Overall, consulting with your healthcare provider ensures that you receive safe, effective, and personalized care tailored to your respiratory health needs. It's an essential step in the decision-making process and can help you navigate the integration of acupuncture or acupressure into your overall healthcare plan.

When considering acupuncture or acupressure for respiratory health or any other condition, it's crucial to be aware of potential allergic reactions and sensitivities. Here's why:

1. **Herbs and Essential Oils**: Some acupuncture treatments may involve the use of herbal remedies or essential oils to enhance therapeutic effects. If you have allergies or sensitivities to certain herbs or oils, it's essential to inform your acupuncturist or acupressure therapist beforehand. They can adjust

the treatment plan to avoid using any substances that may trigger an allergic reaction.

2. **Needle Materials**: Acupuncture needles are typically made of stainless steel, but some practitioners may use needles made of other materials such as gold or silver. If you have metal allergies or sensitivities, it's important to discuss this with your practitioner to ensure that they use needles made of a suitable material.

3. **Skin Sensitivities**: Acupuncture and acupressure involve stimulating specific points on the body, which may cause skin irritation or sensitivities in some individuals. If you have sensitive skin or a history of skin reactions, let your practitioner know so they can adjust the pressure or technique accordingly.

4. **Moxibustion**: Moxibustion is a traditional Chinese medicine technique that involves burning dried mugwort (moxa) near acupuncture points to stimulate healing. If you have allergies or sensitivities to smoke or herbal odors, it's important to discuss this with your practitioner before undergoing moxibustion treatment.

5. **Inhalation Therapies**: Some acupuncture treatments may involve inhalation therapies, such as steam inhalation with herbal blends or essential oils. If you have respiratory allergies or sensitivities, it's crucial to inform your practitioner to avoid any substances that may exacerbate your symptoms.

6. **Patch Testing**: If you're unsure about potential allergies or sensitivities to acupuncture materials or substances used during treatment, your practitioner may recommend a patch test. This involves applying a small amount of the substance to your skin to check for any adverse reactions before proceeding with treatment.

7. **Monitoring**: During acupuncture or acupressure treatment, pay attention to any signs of allergic reactions or sensitivities, such as itching, redness, swelling, or difficulty breathing. If you experience any of these symptoms, inform your practitioner immediately so they can take appropriate action.

By being proactive about discussing allergies and sensitivities with your acupuncturist or acupressure therapist, you can ensure that your treatment is safe and tailored to your individual needs. They can make adjustments to the treatment plan to accommodate any allergies or sensitivities you may have, helping you to experience the benefits of acupuncture or acupressure without any adverse reactions.

Monitoring symptoms is an essential aspect of any treatment plan, including acupuncture or acupressure for respiratory health. Here's why it's important and how to do it effectively:

1. **Assessing Progress**: Monitoring symptoms allows you to track changes in your respiratory condition over time. By regularly assessing your symptoms, you can determine whether acupuncture or acupressure is effectively managing your respiratory symptoms and improving your overall well-being.

2. **Identifying Triggers**: Monitoring symptoms can help you identify potential triggers or exacerbating factors for your respiratory issues. By keeping track of when symptoms occur and any accompanying factors such as environmental conditions or activities, you can pinpoint specific triggers that may contribute to your respiratory symptoms.

3. **Treatment Effectiveness**: Monitoring symptoms allows you to evaluate the effectiveness of acupuncture or acupressure treatment. If you notice improvements in your respiratory symptoms, such as reduced coughing, clearer breathing, or decreased congestion, it indicates that the treatment is working well for you. On the other hand, if your symptoms persist or worsen despite treatment, it may indicate that adjustments to the treatment plan are necessary.

4. **Communication with Practitioner**: By monitoring your symptoms and documenting any changes or patterns, you can provide valuable feedback to your acupuncturist or acupressure therapist. This information enables them to assess your progress, make any necessary modifications to the treatment plan, and provide personalized recommendations for managing your respiratory health.

5. **Tracking Trends**: Monitoring symptoms over time allows you to identify trends or patterns in your respiratory condition. For example, you may notice seasonal variations in your symptoms or specific triggers that consistently exacerbate your respiratory issues. Understanding these patterns

can help you develop strategies to manage your condition more effectively.

6. **Adjusting Lifestyle**: Monitoring symptoms can also help you make informed decisions about lifestyle modifications or self-care practices that may benefit your respiratory health. For example, if you notice that certain activities or environmental factors worsen your symptoms, you can take steps to avoid or minimize exposure to these triggers.

To effectively monitor your symptoms, consider the following tips:

- Keep a symptom journal or diary to record details such as the frequency, severity, and duration of your respiratory symptoms.
- Note any factors that may influence your symptoms, such as exposure to allergens, changes in weather, or stress levels.
- Use rating scales or subjective assessments to quantify the intensity of your symptoms, such as a numerical scale from 0 to 10 or descriptive terms like mild, moderate, or severe.
- Be consistent and diligent in tracking your symptoms, recording information regularly and accurately to provide a comprehensive picture of your respiratory health.

By actively monitoring your symptoms and communicating with your practitioner, you can optimize the effectiveness of acupuncture or acupressure treatment for respiratory health and make informed decisions about managing your condition.

Integrating acupuncture or acupressure with conventional treatment for respiratory conditions can offer a comprehensive approach to managing your health. Here's how you can effectively integrate these alternative therapies with conventional treatments:

1. **Consultation with Healthcare Provider**: Before incorporating acupuncture or acupressure into your treatment plan, consult with your primary healthcare provider or specialist. They can provide guidance on how these alternative therapies may complement your conventional treatment and ensure that there are no contraindications or interactions with your current medications or therapies.

2. **Collaboration between Practitioners**: Encourage open communication and collaboration between your acupuncturist or acupressure

therapist and your conventional healthcare providers. This allows for coordinated care and ensures that all healthcare providers are aware of your treatment plan and can provide support and guidance as needed.

3. **Understanding Treatment Goals**: Clearly define your treatment goals and expectations with both your conventional healthcare providers and your alternative therapy practitioner. Discuss how acupuncture or acupressure can support your overall health and well-being, as well as specific goals related to managing your respiratory condition.

4. **Comprehensive Assessment**: Work with your healthcare team to conduct a comprehensive assessment of your respiratory health, including diagnostic tests, medical history review, and evaluation of symptoms. This helps identify areas where acupuncture or acupressure may provide additional support or symptom relief.

5. **Treatment Plan Integration**: Integrate acupuncture or acupressure sessions into your overall treatment plan in collaboration with your healthcare providers. This may involve scheduling sessions between conventional treatments,

incorporating them as adjunct therapies, or alternating between different modalities based on your needs and response to treatment.

6. **Monitoring and Evaluation**: Regularly monitor your respiratory symptoms and overall health status to evaluate the effectiveness of integrated treatment. Keep your healthcare providers informed of any changes or improvements in your symptoms, as well as any concerns or challenges you may encounter during treatment.

7. **Individualized Approach**: Recognize that integrative treatment is personalized and may vary depending on your unique health needs, preferences, and response to therapy. Your healthcare team can tailor the treatment plan to address your specific respiratory condition and optimize outcomes.

8. **Patient Education**: Take an active role in educating yourself about both conventional treatments and alternative therapies like acupuncture or acupressure. Understand how these treatments work, their potential benefits and limitations, and what to expect during sessions.

9. **Holistic Wellness**: Emphasize the importance of holistic wellness and self-care practices alongside conventional and alternative treatments. This may include lifestyle modifications, stress management techniques, dietary changes, and exercise routines that support respiratory health and overall well-being.

By integrating acupuncture or acupressure with conventional treatment for respiratory conditions, you can access a broader range of therapeutic options and potentially enhance the effectiveness of your overall treatment plan. Collaboration between healthcare providers and a patient-centered approach can help you achieve optimal respiratory health outcomes and improve your quality of life.

Conclusion

In conclusion, respiratory conditions such as pneumonia and asthma can significantly impact an individual's quality of life, requiring comprehensive management strategies for effective relief and long-term wellness. While conventional treatments play a crucial role in managing these conditions, integrating alternative therapies like acupuncture and acupressure can offer additional support and symptom relief.

Throughout this guide, we've explored various aspects of pneumonia and asthma, including their understanding, differentiation, and the importance of natural remedies. Lifestyle changes, dietary modifications, exercise, environmental adjustments, stress management techniques, and herbal remedies are all integral components of holistic respiratory care. Furthermore, we've delved into specific natural remedies such as essential oils, homeopathic remedies, dietary supplements, breathing exercises, steam therapy, and acupuncture/acupressure points for respiratory health.

However, it's essential to approach these treatments with caution, consulting with healthcare providers and ensuring personalized, integrated care tailored to individual needs and preferences. Monitoring symptoms, collaborating between healthcare practitioners, and emphasizing holistic wellness are crucial for optimizing outcomes and achieving sustainable respiratory health.

By combining conventional treatments with alternative therapies in a comprehensive, patient-centered approach, individuals can effectively manage respiratory conditions, alleviate symptoms, and improve overall well-being. With proper guidance, education, and self-care practices, individuals can empower themselves to lead healthier lives and enjoy greater respiratory comfort and vitality.

Here's a recap of the natural remedies discussed for pneumonia and asthma:

1. **Herbal Remedies**:
    - Eucalyptus
    - Ginger
    - Turmeric
    - Licorice Root
    - Ginseng

2. **Essential Oils for Respiratory Health**:
   - Peppermint Oil
   - Tea Tree Oil
   - Lavender Oil
   - Eucalyptus Oil
   - Oregano Oil

3. **Homeopathic Remedies**:
   - Antimonium Tartaricum
   - Arsenicum Album
   - Bryonia
   - Ipecacuanha
   - Spongia Tosta

4. **Dietary Supplements**:
   - Vitamin C
   - Vitamin D
   - Magnesium
   - Omega-3 Fatty Acids
   - Quercetin

5. **Breathing Exercises and Techniques**:
   - Diaphragmatic Breathing
   - Pursed Lip Breathing
   - Buteyko Breathing Technique
   - Yoga and Pranayama

6. **Steam Therapy and Humidification**:
   - Steam Inhalation
   - Humidifiers and Vaporizers
   - Herbal Steam Blends

7. **Acupuncture and Acupressure Points**:
   - Lung Meridian Points
   - Conception Vessel Meridian Points
   - Governing Vessel Meridian Points

These natural remedies offer various benefits for respiratory health, including reducing inflammation, supporting immune function, promoting relaxation, and improving respiratory function. However, it's important to use them under the guidance of healthcare professionals and integrate them into a comprehensive treatment plan tailored to individual needs.

The importance of a personalized approach to managing respiratory conditions like pneumonia and asthma cannot be overstated. Here's why it's crucial:

1. **Individual Variability**: Each person's experience with respiratory conditions can vary widely based on factors such as the underlying

cause, severity of symptoms, medical history, lifestyle, and environmental factors. A personalized approach takes these individual differences into account and tailors treatment to meet specific needs.

2. **Targeted Treatment**: Personalized care allows healthcare providers to target treatment interventions to address the unique needs and preferences of each individual. This targeted approach increases the likelihood of treatment effectiveness and reduces the risk of adverse effects or complications.

3. **Optimized Outcomes**: By considering the individual characteristics and circumstances of each patient, personalized care aims to optimize treatment outcomes and improve overall health and well-being. It allows healthcare providers to adjust treatment plans as needed based on patient responses and evolving health needs.

4. **Patient-Centered Care**: Personalized care places the patient at the center of the healthcare experience, empowering them to actively participate in decision-making and self-management. It takes into account patients' values, preferences, and goals, fostering a

collaborative relationship between patients and healthcare providers.

5. **Holistic Approach**: A personalized approach to respiratory care considers not only the physical symptoms but also the psychological, social, and environmental factors that may influence health and well-being. It emphasizes holistic wellness and addresses the interconnectedness of body, mind, and spirit.

6. **Improved Adherence**: Tailoring treatment to individual needs and preferences can enhance patient satisfaction and adherence to treatment plans. Patients are more likely to follow recommendations and engage in self-care practices when they feel heard, understood, and actively involved in their care.

7. **Prevention and Wellness Promotion**: Personalized care extends beyond symptom management to include preventive measures and wellness promotion strategies. By identifying individual risk factors and health goals, healthcare providers can offer targeted interventions to prevent exacerbations, minimize complications, and promote long-term respiratory health.

In summary, a personalized approach to managing respiratory conditions recognizes the uniqueness of each individual and seeks to provide tailored treatment interventions that address their specific needs, preferences, and circumstances. By embracing personalized care, healthcare providers can optimize treatment outcomes, enhance patient engagement and satisfaction, and promote holistic well-being.

Long-term management strategies for respiratory conditions such as pneumonia and asthma focus on controlling symptoms, preventing exacerbations, and promoting overall respiratory health and well-being. Here are some key components of long-term management:

1. **Medication Management**: Work with your healthcare provider to develop a comprehensive medication regimen tailored to your specific respiratory condition. This may include bronchodilators, corticosteroids, antibiotics (for pneumonia), and other medications to manage symptoms and prevent flare-ups.

2. **Lifestyle Modifications**: Adopt healthy lifestyle habits that support respiratory health, such

as maintaining a balanced diet, staying hydrated, getting regular exercise, avoiding smoking and exposure to secondhand smoke, and managing stress effectively.

3. **Environmental Control**: Identify and minimize exposure to environmental triggers that can exacerbate respiratory symptoms, such as allergens, pollutants, and respiratory irritants. Use air purifiers, allergen-proof bedding, and proper ventilation to create a clean and healthy indoor environment.

4. **Allergy Management**: If allergies contribute to your respiratory symptoms, work with an allergist to identify specific allergens and develop an allergy management plan. This may include allergen avoidance strategies, allergy medications, immunotherapy (allergy shots), and other interventions to reduce allergic reactions.

5. **Regular Monitoring and Follow-up**: Stay vigilant about monitoring your respiratory symptoms and seek prompt medical attention if you experience any changes or worsening of symptoms. Attend regular follow-up appointments with your healthcare provider to assess your respiratory

function, adjust treatment as needed, and address any concerns or questions.

6. **Self-Management Education**: Educate yourself about your respiratory condition, including its causes, triggers, symptoms, and treatment options. Learn how to recognize early warning signs of exacerbations and how to respond appropriately. Participate in self-management programs or support groups to gain valuable skills and support for managing your condition effectively.

7. **Respiratory Rehabilitation**: Consider participating in a pulmonary rehabilitation program tailored to individuals with chronic respiratory conditions. These programs typically include exercise training, education, breathing exercises, and psychosocial support to improve respiratory function, enhance quality of life, and reduce disability.

8. **Complementary and Alternative Therapies**: Explore complementary and alternative therapies such as acupuncture, acupressure, herbal remedies, breathing exercises, and relaxation techniques to complement conventional treatments and promote respiratory health. Consult with your healthcare provider

before trying any new therapies to ensure their safety and effectiveness.

9. **Emergency Preparedness**: Develop an emergency action plan in collaboration with your healthcare provider to outline steps to take in the event of a respiratory emergency or exacerbation. Ensure that you have access to rescue medications, emergency contacts, and medical information to facilitate timely intervention and treatment.

By implementing these long-term management strategies, individuals with respiratory conditions can effectively control symptoms, minimize exacerbations, and maintain optimal respiratory health and quality of life over the long term. Consistent adherence to treatment plans, proactive self-management, and ongoing communication with healthcare providers are essential for achieving optimal outcomes and maximizing well-being.

www.ingramcontent.com/pod-product-compliance
Lightning Source LLC
Chambersburg PA
CBHW052201220526
45471CB00004B/1767